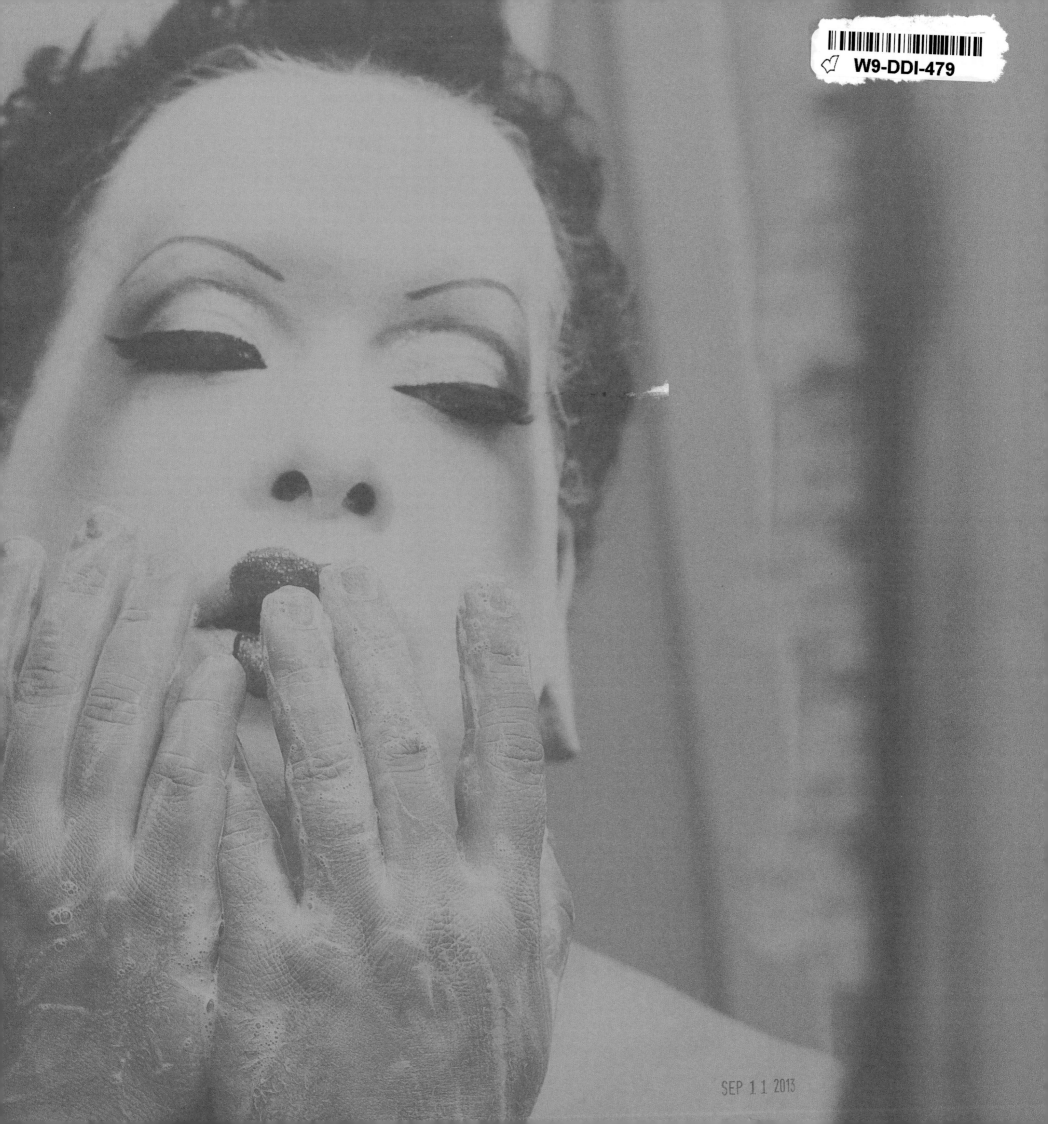

GETTING INTO FACE

52 Mondays featuring JoJo Baby and Sal-E

BERNARD COLBERT

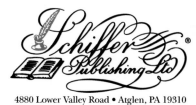

4880 Lower Valley Road • Atglen, PA 19310

Copyright © 2012 by Bernard Colbert

Library of Congress Control Number: 2012937359

Designed by Justin Watkinson
Type set in Futura Std

ISBN: 978-0-7643-4201-1
Printed in China

Published by Schiffer Publishing Ltd.
4880 Lower Valley Road
Atglen, PA 19310
Phone: (610) 593-1777; Fax: (610) 593-2002
E-mail: Info@schifferbooks.com

For the largest selection of fine reference books on this and related subjects, please visit our website at **www.schifferbooks.com.** You may also write for a free catalog.

This book may be purchased from the publisher.
Please try your bookstore first.

We are always looking for people to write books on new and related subjects.
If you have an idea for a book, please contact us at proposals@schifferbooks.com

Schiffer Books are available at special discounts for bulk purchases for sales promotions or premiums. Special editions, including personalized covers, corporate imprints, and excerpts can be created in large quantities for special needs. For more information contact the publisher.

In Europe, Schiffer books are distributed by
Bushwood Books
6 Marksbury Ave.
Kew Gardens
Surrey TW9 4JF England
Phone: 44 (0) 20 8392 8585; Fax: 44 (0) 20 8392 9876
E-mail: info@bushwoodbooks.co.uk
Website: www.bushwoodbooks.co.uk

This book is dedicated to three very special women:

JoJo's mother, Sal's mother, and my mother.

Also, to my brother, whom I miss very much.

"Ich Bin Kunst" ("I Am Art")

This is a song written and performed by
Boy George as a tribute to Leigh Bowery,
featured in the 2002 stage musical production *Taboo*.

CONTENTS

Post Warhol superstar but pre reality TV show celebrity, a new structure for fame solidified. With its roots in such voyeuristic cultural phenomenon as the pansy craze of the 1930s and the Harlem ball scene, the fame tag "club kid" came into focus in the 1990s, and JoJo Baby is one of its pioneers and remains one of its super novas.

Club kids are nightclub denizens and rose to commodified fame due to the existence of mega clubs needing to bring in large numbers of patrons to fill their cavernous square footage. The club kid dressed as outrageously as possible and brought a general circus like atmosphere. Club kid style explodes traditional notions of gender-appropriate clothing as well as any notion of what might constitute clothing, accessories, makeup, or hair. To truly stand out in this hyper-imaginative demi-monde you must truly be creative, talented, and beyond the beyond. As with many other professions, it also helps to have a good personality. JoJo Baby is just such a standout flaming creature.

But JoJo Baby, a pet name his mother called him as a child, is so much more than a club kid. An accomplished multi-media artist from Polaroid collages to oil paintings, JoJo has also created hair and makeup for numerous stage productions, artists, and celebrity clients including the Chicago Bull's Dennis Rodman's infamous hair color treatments. JoJo is perhaps best known, however, as a doll maker. Working side by side for many years with famed dollsmith Greer Lankton (1958–1996), JoJo meticulously creates full armature figures brimming with personality, whimsy, and elegance.

Looking at JoJo's striking dolls that bring to mind influences as diverse as Jim Henson (1936–1990) and Clive Barker, and range in size from a few inches tall to close to ten feet tall, it is tempting to think of his dressing up as some sort of extension or transference onto his own body of his doll-making practice. Certainly, he masterfully uses many of the same skill sets as he shapes and encrusts his body and face with all sorts of found, at hand, or inexpensive materials to become a living sculpture.

Bernard Colbert's *Getting into Face* gathers photographs of JoJo Baby and Sal-E, his clubbing companion. Sal-E likewise brings strong skill sets in hair, makeup, and costume to the game, and together the dynamic shape-shifting duo have ruled Chicago nightclubs, including the Boom Boom Room, for ten plus years. Their living art has seen them transform into every type of thing and being from psychedelic Hindi gods to comic book villains. Whether their creations are light or dark, spiritual or pop, JoJo and Sal-E pair, complement, and bounce off each other.

The photographer and body artists share studios in the same Chicago building, the Flatiron Building in the Wicker Park neighborhood, and struck up a friendship. Colbert soon began taking a few shots of JoJo and Sal-E each night before they ventured out in their fantastic creations. Over the course of five years, Colbert created the body of work represented here. In some ways the collaboration brings to mind Fergus Greer's photographic studio studies of Leigh Bowery (1961–1994), JoJo and Sal-E's British counterpart.

Colbert's portraits were mainly shot in the Flatiron building against generic architectural backgrounds yet every now and then a piece of tin ceiling, stair rail, or window frame stands out. Working independently, Colbert planned the night's photo staging area without prior knowledge of what JoJo and Sal-E might be sporting. The color images are mainly waist up and focus on the elaborately made-up faces. A few are full body, stressing more the costume or pose. A few show JoJo and Sal-E in non-voids and recontextualize them in and against specific environments like in the street or a late-night restaurant. The nightclub, the club kids' natural environment, is generally not a setting for Colbert's work. Under his more tightly controlled studio environments, Colbert's rigorous images compel a closer scrutiny of JoJo and Sal-E's flawless looks. The pictures capture them at their just-out-of-the-dressing-room freshest and a sense of wide-eyed anticipation for the long night ahead is clearly evident as is a divide-and-conquer attitude. The subjects display ultimate confidence, showing no doubt they are beautiful and fantastic.

Colbert's colorful photos more than rise to the challenge of capturing the surface image two equally creative and colorful subjects create and present. The photos also reveal some of the truths behind the elaborate masks of makeup and costume. Both photographic objects and living subjects are high art.

—Joe E. Jeffreys

Joe E. Jeffreys is a drag historian. He produces *Drag Show Video Vérité* and his video work has screened at film festivals worldwide and museums including MOMA and the Tate Modern.

Getting into Face is a portfolio of digital photographs documenting the work of two performance artists, JoJo Baby and Sal-E, over a period of 5 years, beginning in 2007.

JoJo and Sal have dedicated their lives to reinventing themselves on a daily basis.

Call them what you will, but they are *artists*—and their bodies and their lives are their canvas. Watch them as they execute their craft with masterful precision.

To those of you who are weak at heart, be cautioned. The images contained within this book might just lift your spirits too much for you to bear.

If you aren't afraid to laugh or to smile, (especially at yourself), feel free to turn the page and enter their world. Enjoy!

ACKNOWLEDGMENTS

Special thanks to all our many fans who have kept me going with their joyful enthusiasm, especially:

My Family: Michael, Laura, Claire, Marc, and Brandon.

My supporters: Andrea and Dick Ginsburg; Annette and Phil of "Eye Want;" Patricia Billings; Leslie Ramirez; Stacey Weber; the Flat Iron Artist Association artists; Steve Hamada; Peter Hernandez; Nick Azzaro; John Gregg; Allan Shiffrin; Ken Willow and the rest of the Core3Creative crew, past and present; Clive Barker; Mark Danforth; Dana Bruning; Eric Downey; Abel Beruman; Joseph and Tomoko Nagle; Ray Beckley; Jeff Jenkins; and Robert Preston Coddington.

This project is partially supported by a Community Arts Assistance Program grant from the City of Chicago Department of Cultural Affairs and the Illinois Arts Council, a state agency.

I first met JoJo Baby when I first moved into the Flat Iron arts building of Wicker Park, Chicago, in the fall of 2002. As a commercial photographer, I had always wanted to venture into fine-art photography. I had been waiting to find a subject matter which I felt was worthy.

As JoJo's neighbor, I quickly became one of JoJo and Sal's most avid admirers. Although I was intimidated to approach them at first, I eventually asked if they would grant me access to their world and for the honor of photographing them.

Luckily for me, JoJo and Sal love the camera and the limelight. They don't go out in public dressed the way they do hoping to go unnoticed.

I discovered that Monday nights were the best night to catch JoJo and his partner in crime, Sal-E.

JoJo and Sal work various nightclubs, anniversaries, and parties, sometimes together, sometimes apart, but for about 20 years, JoJo and (eventually) Sal have worked at the Boom Boom Room, the longest running house music night in the world. Boom Boom Room is also Industry Night and Gay Night, hosted (at the time of this writing) at Green Dolphin Street in Chicago.

Things at the club get going at around midnight.

JoJo and Sal are supposed to be at work by 11 P.M. Truth is they are at my studio being photographed from about 10:45 until 11:03 because we are having way too much fun taking pictures.

Yes, JoJo Baby is his legal name. As his friends like to say, "That's Mr. Baby to you!" Let me introduce him to you and he will be "your JoJo," as well as mine, for ever more.

Sometimes they are superheroes, sometimes super villains, they are always the tricksters.

When I first decided to create this series of images, I had one broad reaching decision to make.

I could have defined the project as "JoJo Baby and friends," and sought out each of the many wonderful and colorful club kids who JoJo and Sal-E both know. I also could have done a book called *JoJo Baby*, since there is certainly enough depth and interest there to deserve an exclusive treatment.

After having known JoJo and Sal-E for a couple of years, and especially while working together, I became aware of (and somewhat in awe of) their very special friendship.

These two amazingly talented individuals—who are incredibly competitive—tirelessly, ceaselessly, push each other (and themselves) to increasing heights, but always with such great respect and mutual admiration.

I see a bond there stronger than a brother's love and a sibling rivalry. I see a very unique bond which is transcendent and is more positive, supportive, and nurturing than a romantic love.

To me, that is very much the story here.

One art critic wrote that they work so well together because Sal-E is a perfect "Robin" to JoJo's "Batman." Great praise to both men, I think. Although Sal-E is second to no one, when it comes to JoJo, Sal seems very much honored to play *his* "Robin."

To JoJo and Sal, from my heart, thank you for entertaining and inspiring me all of these years.

Cheers,
Bernard

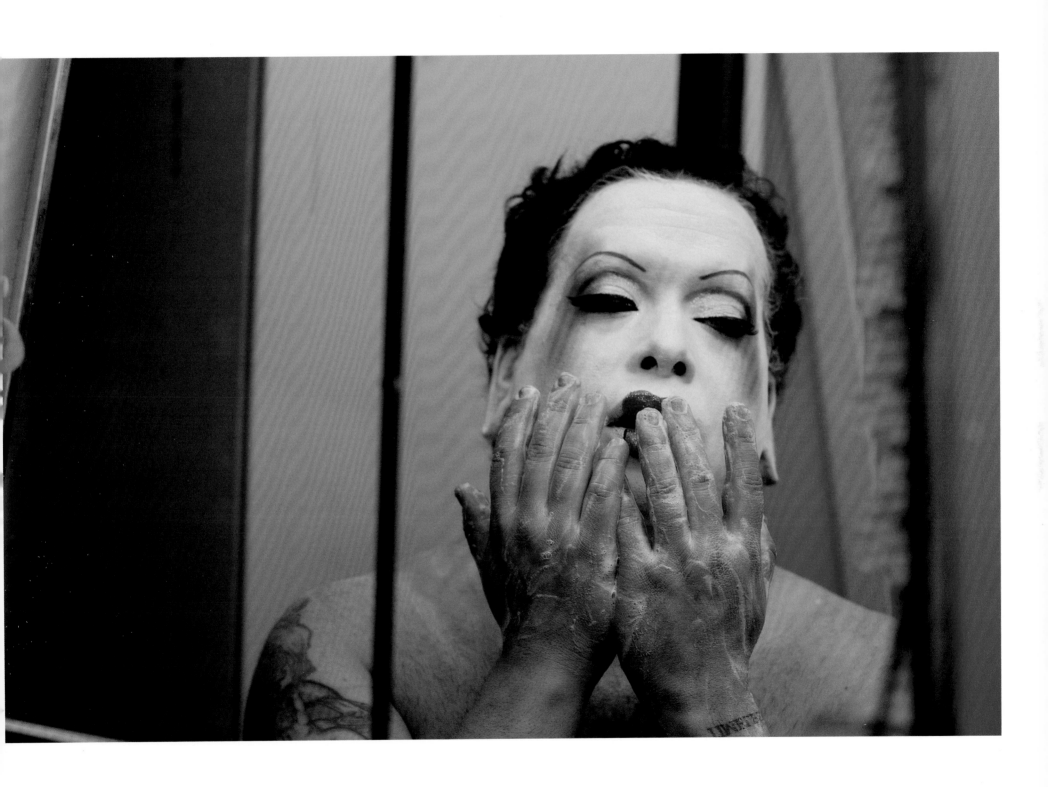

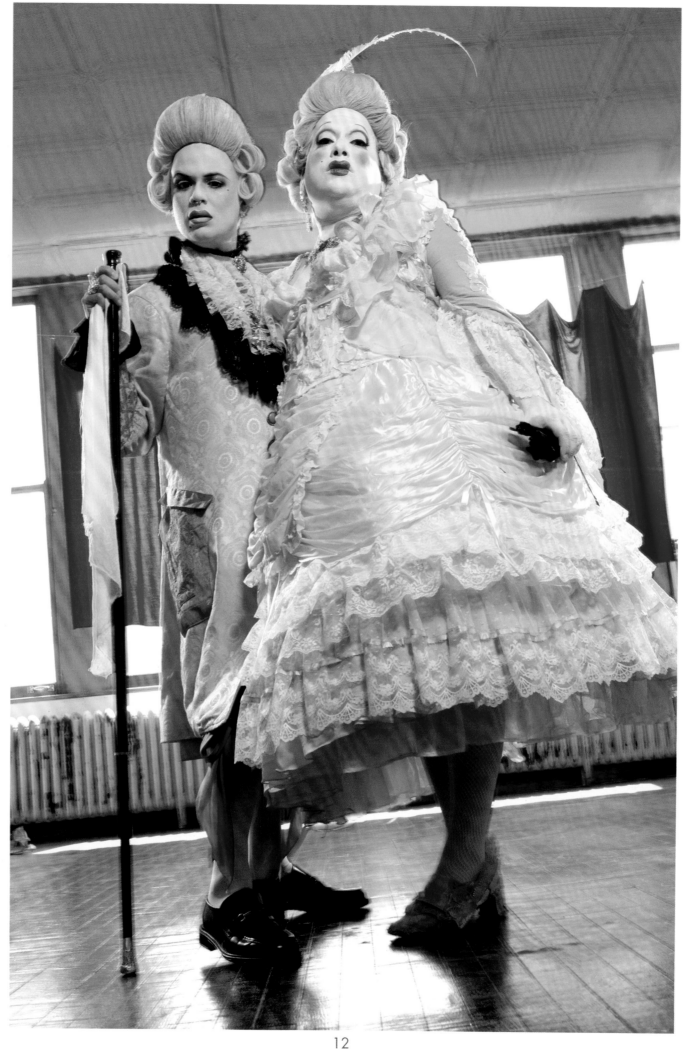

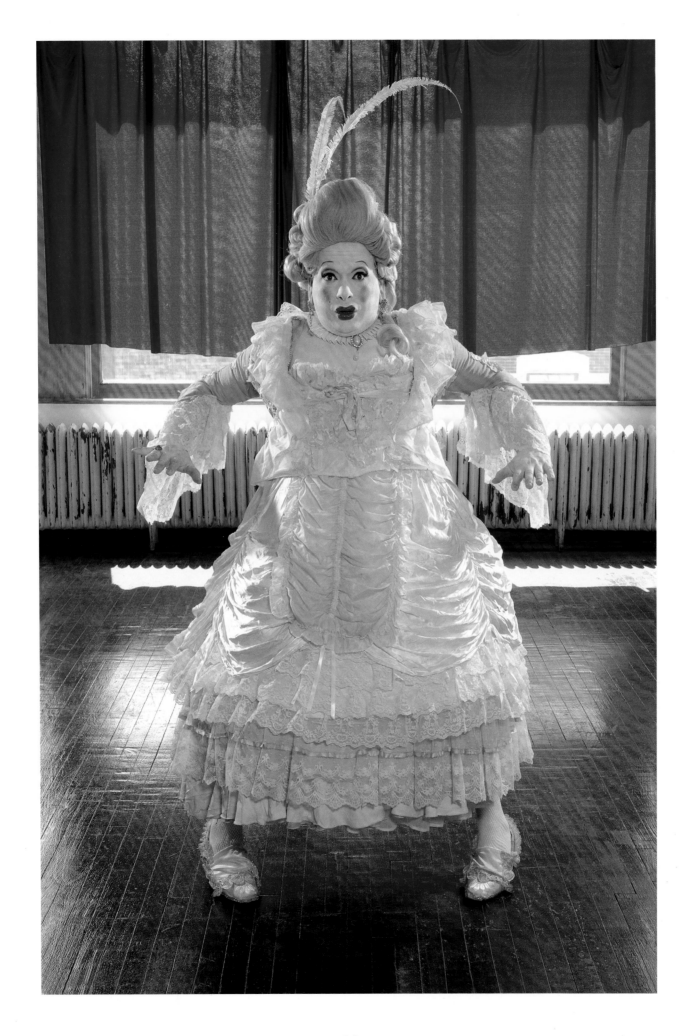

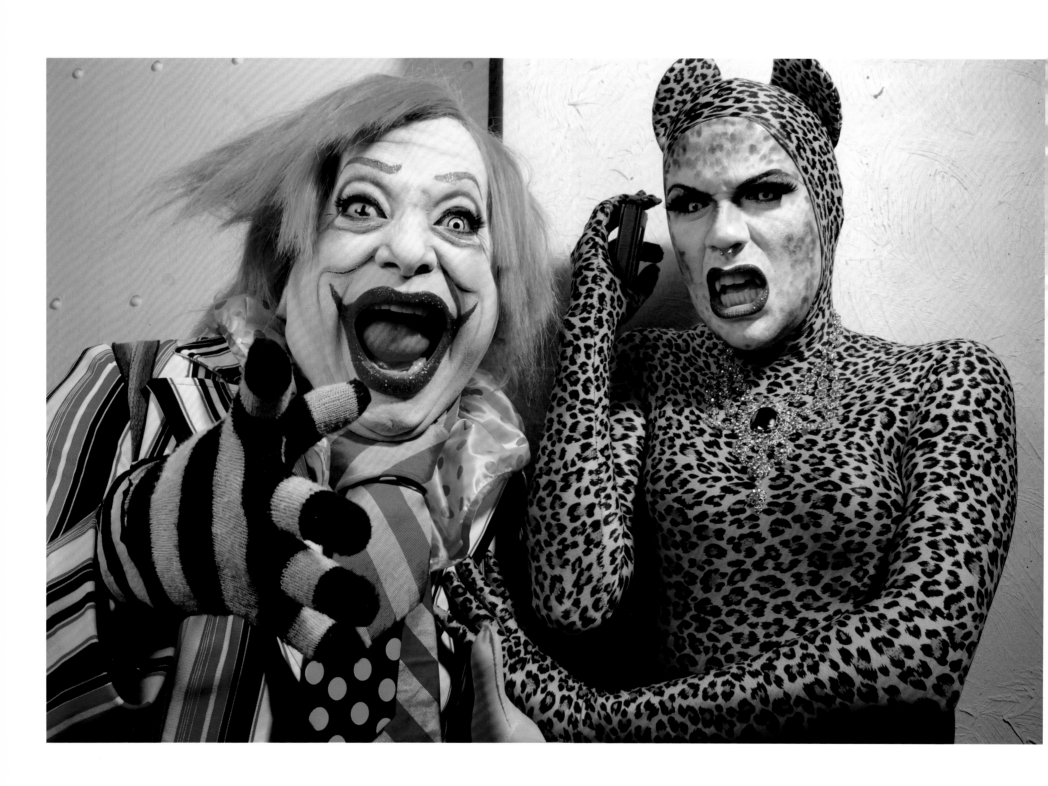

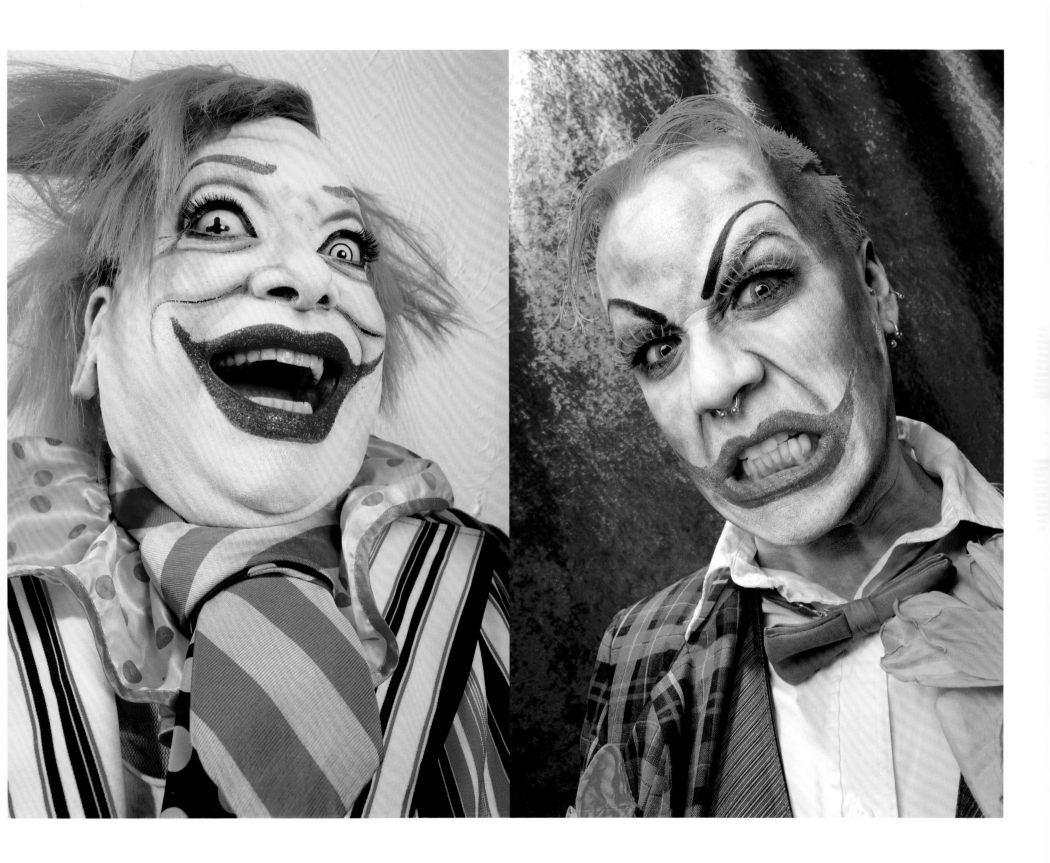

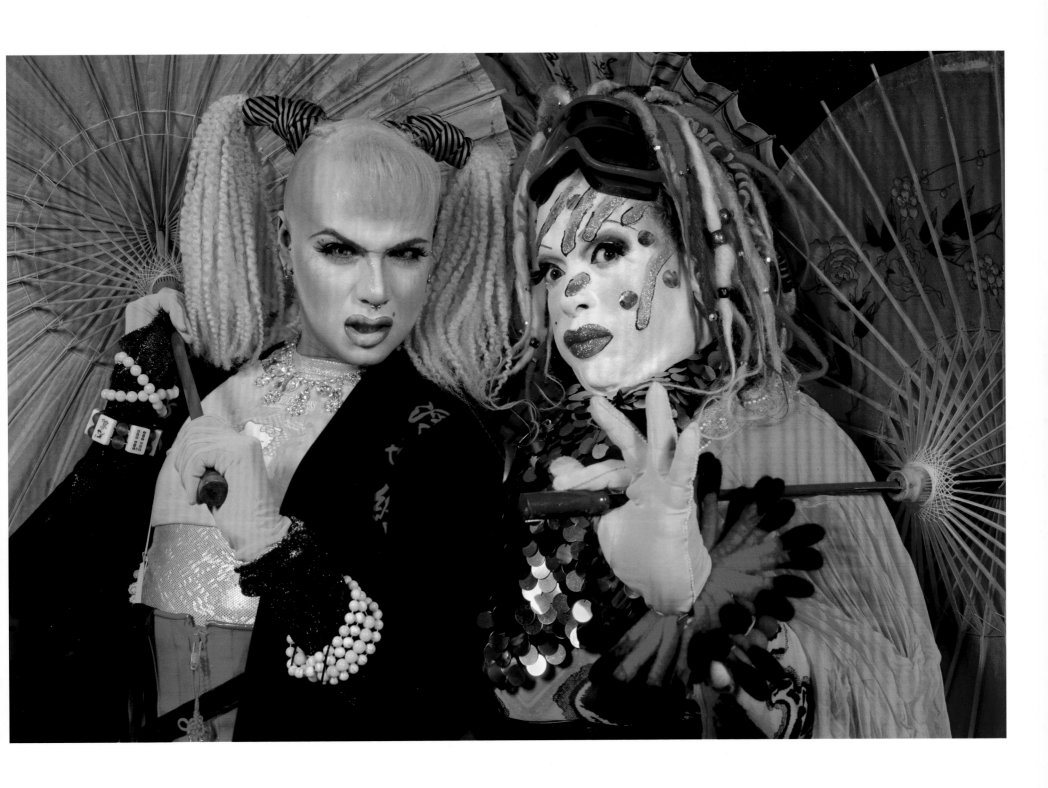

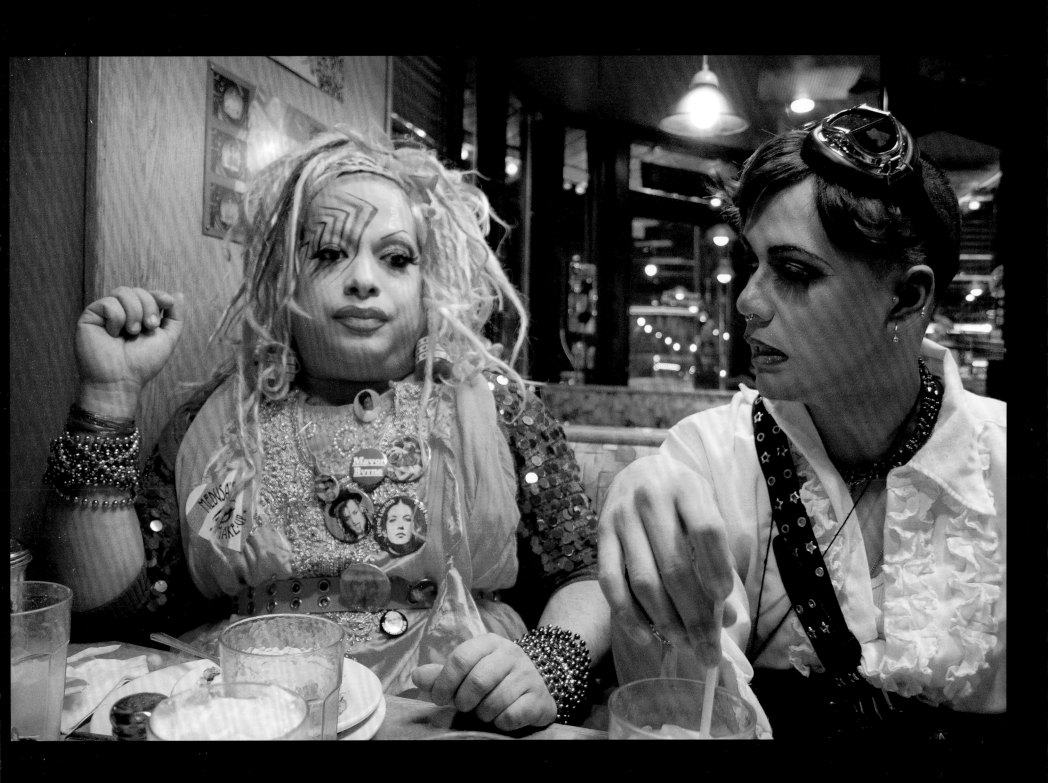

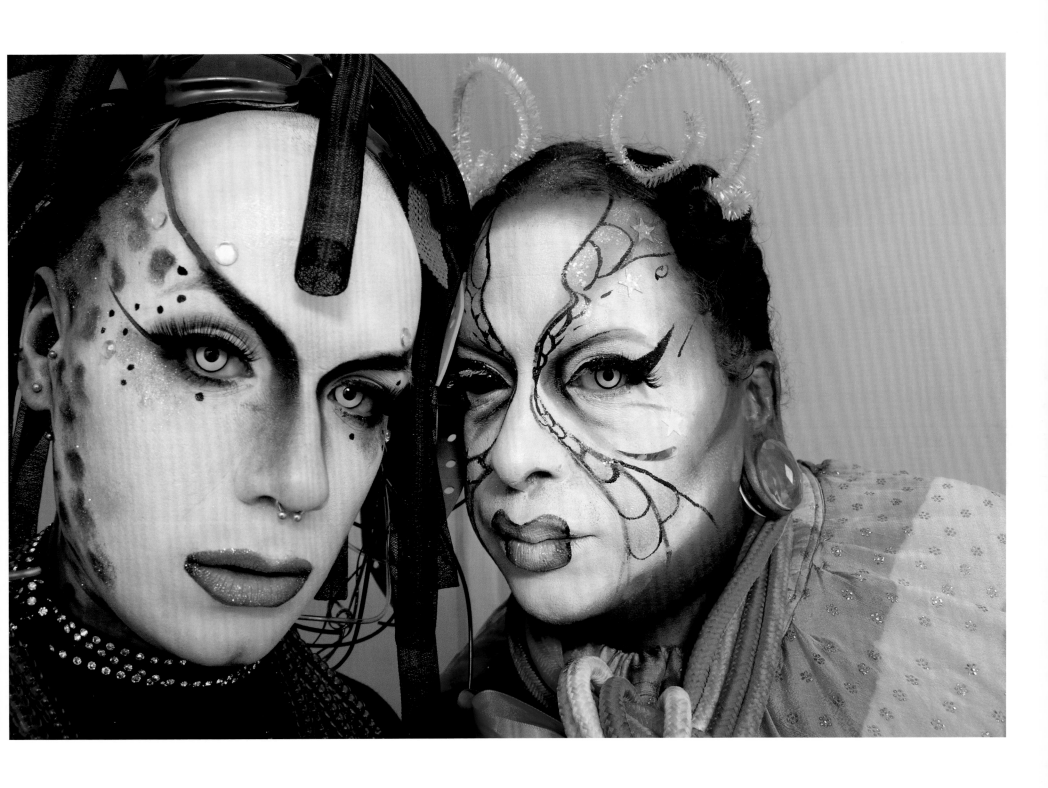

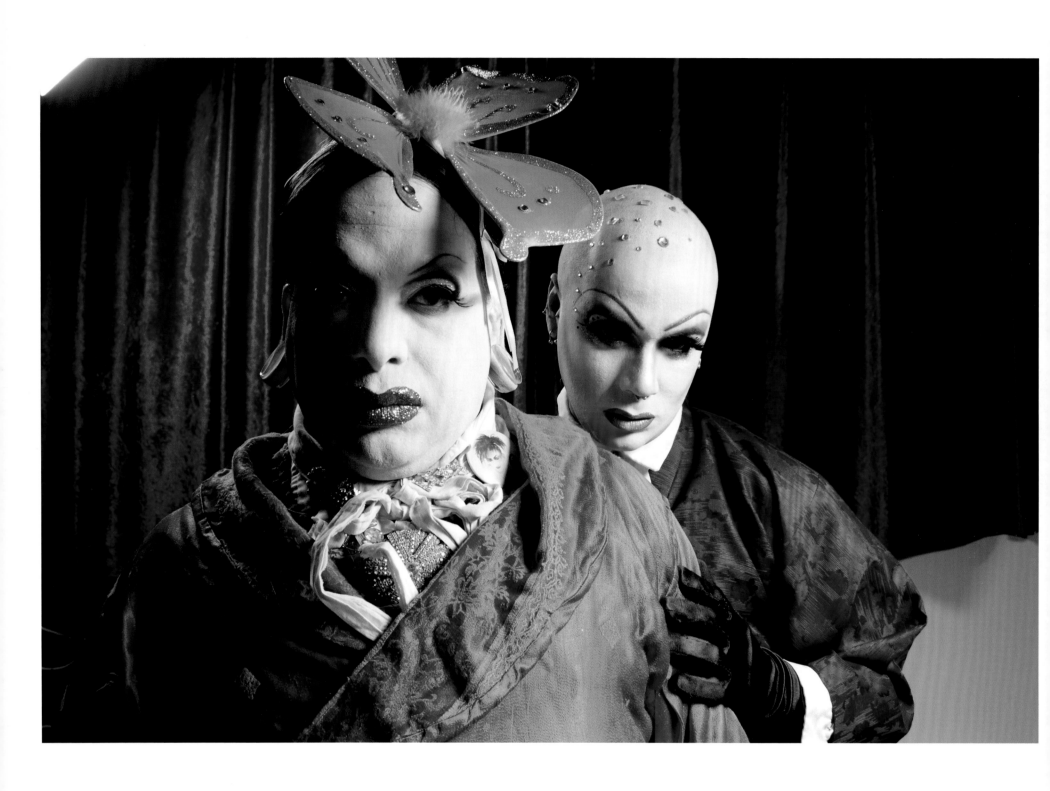

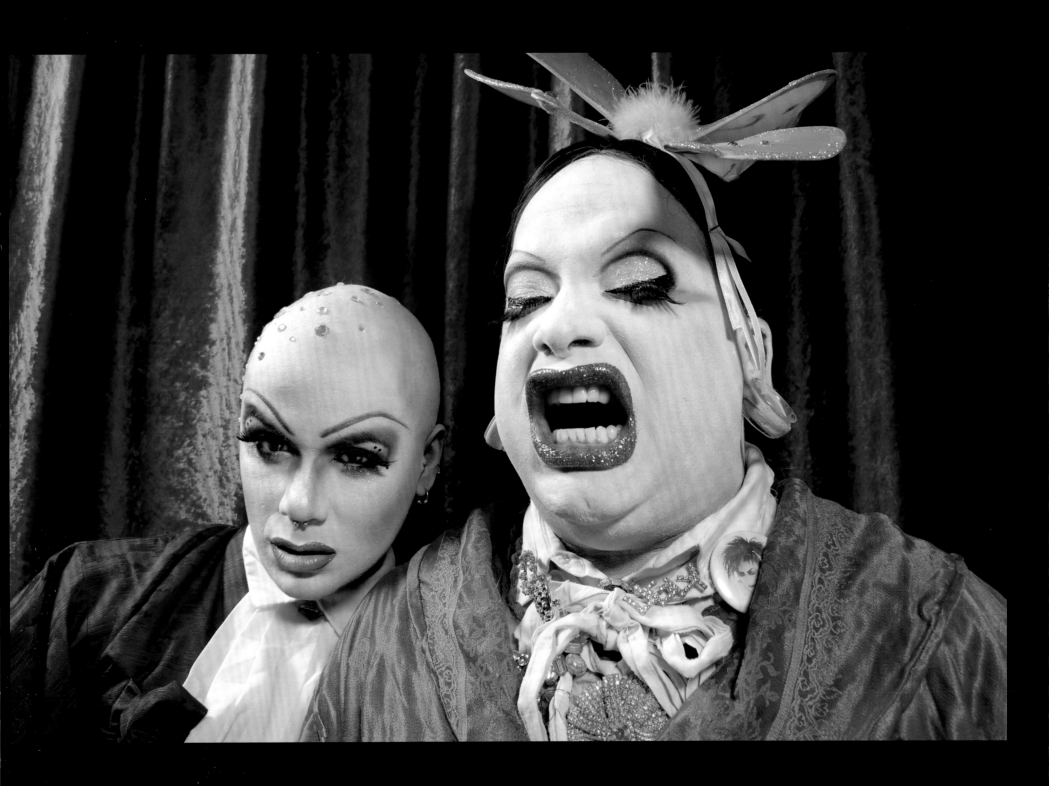

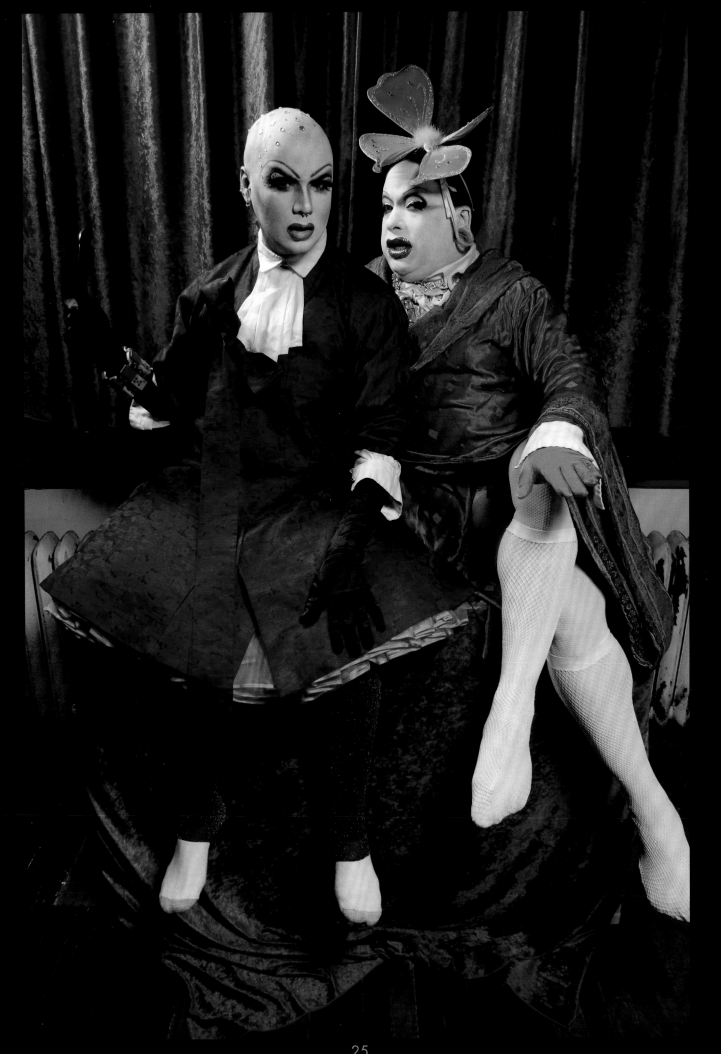

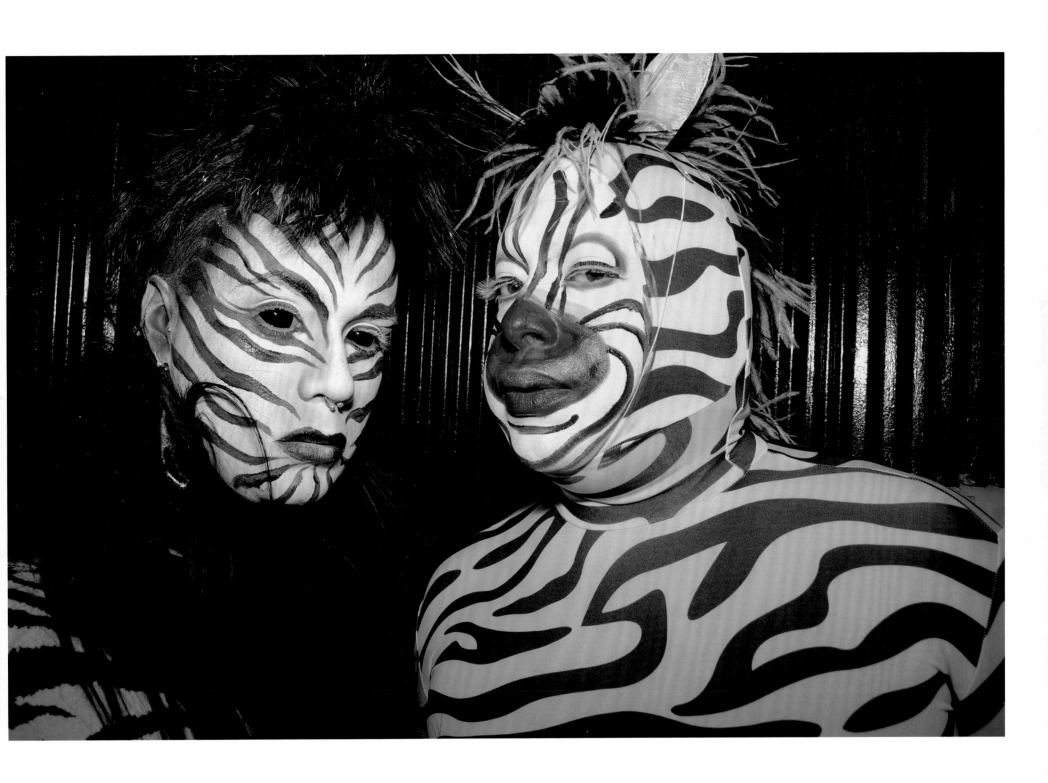

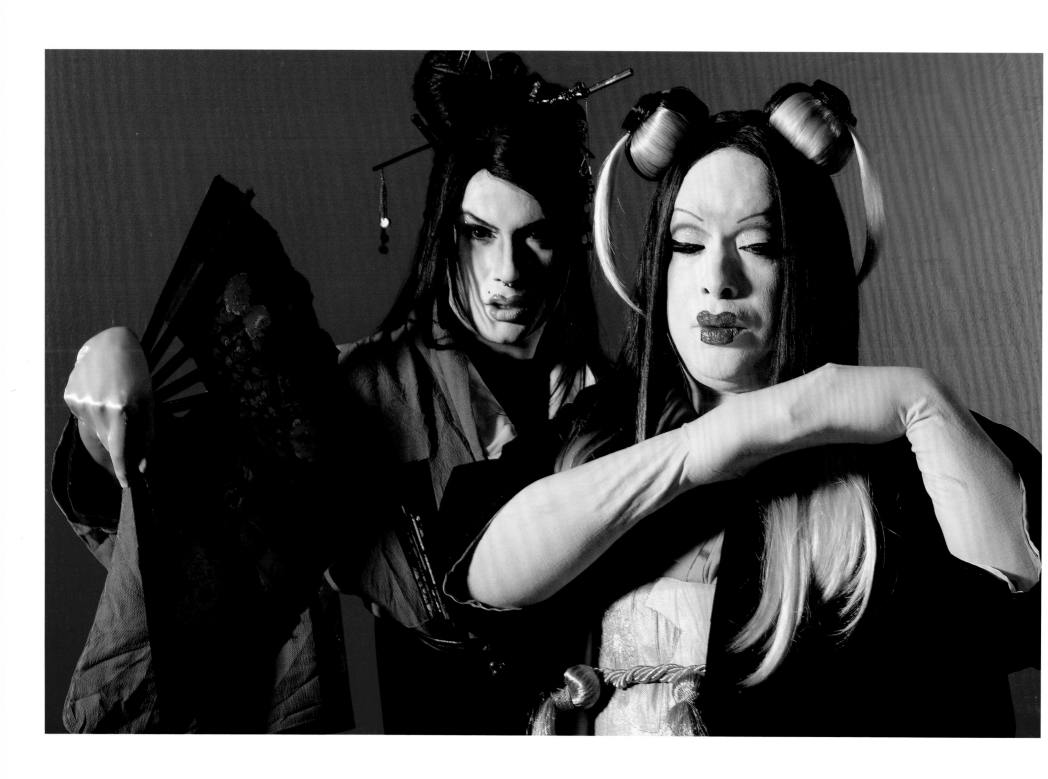

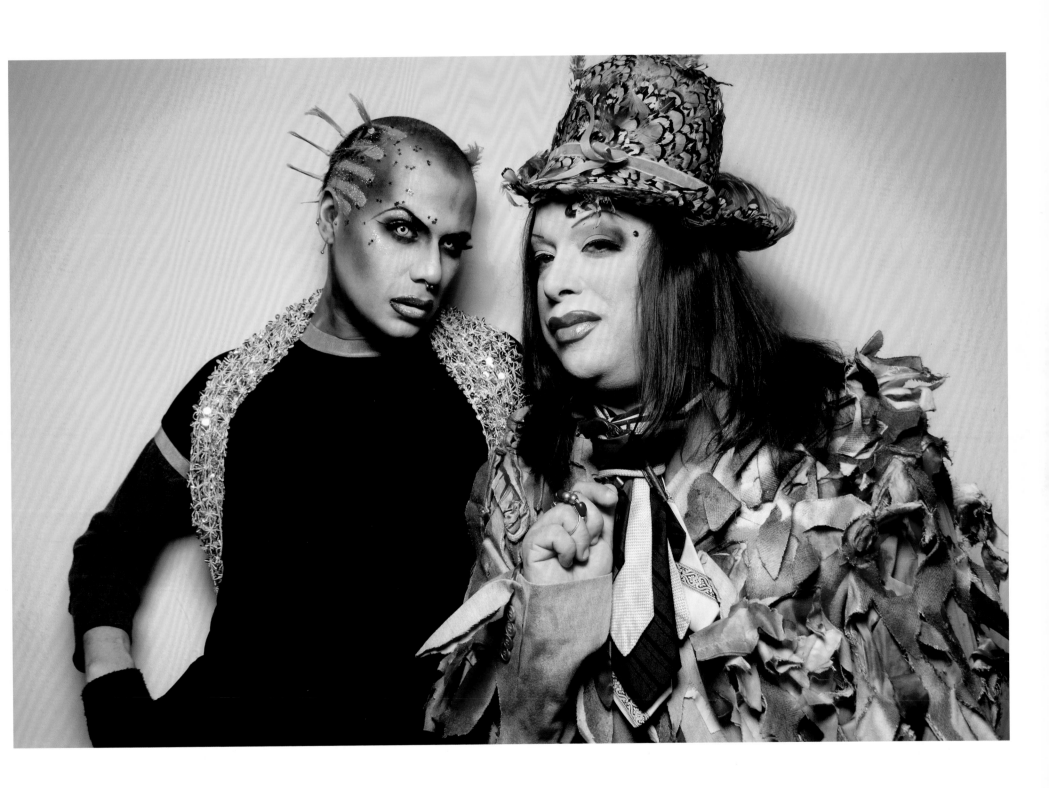

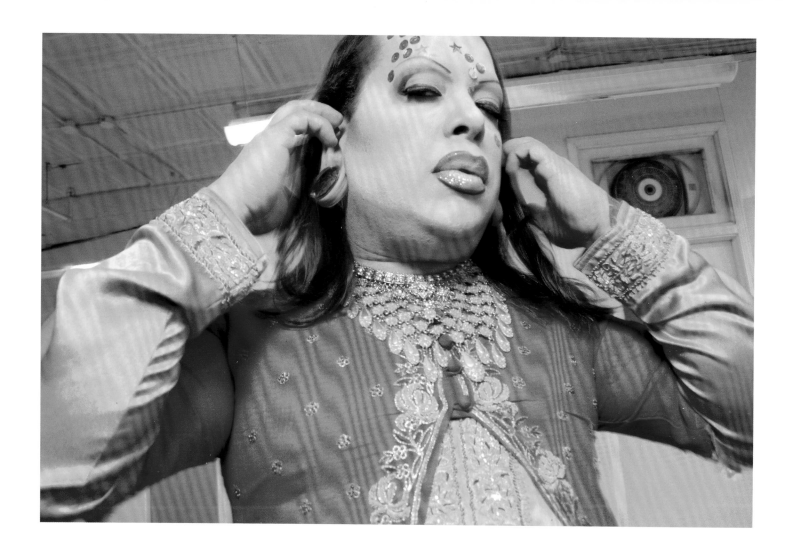

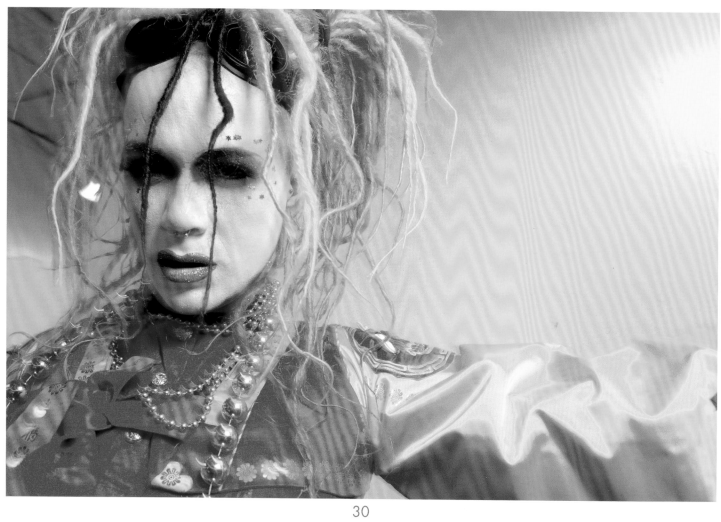

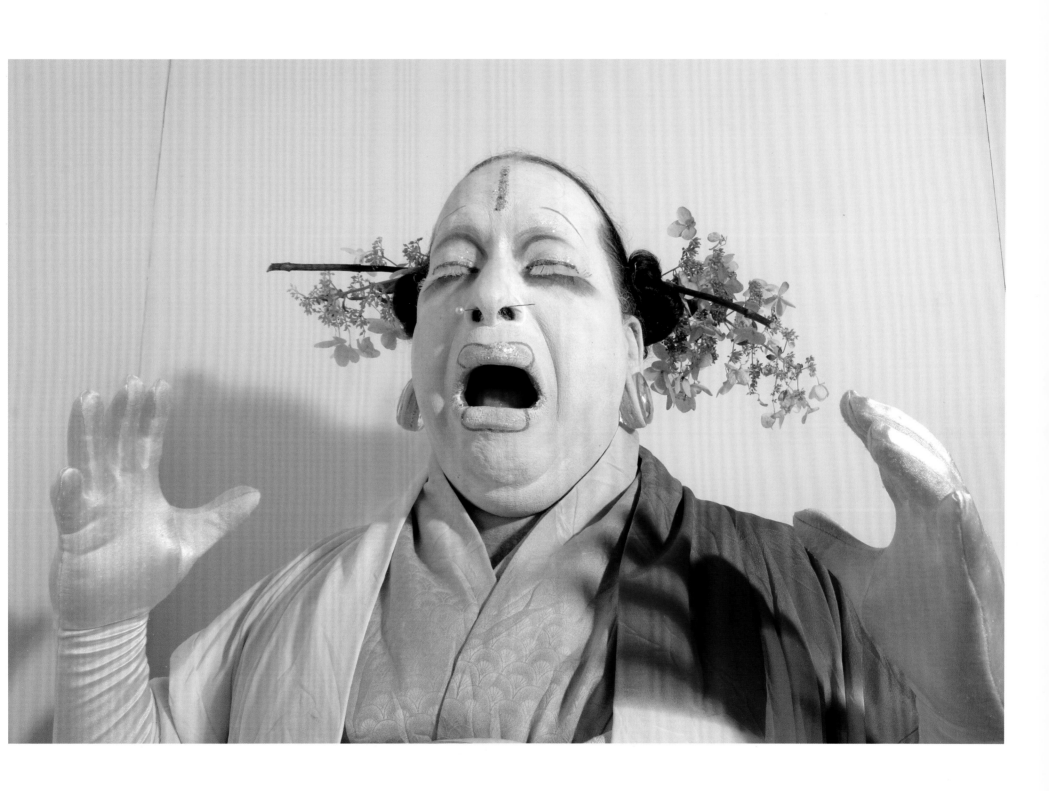

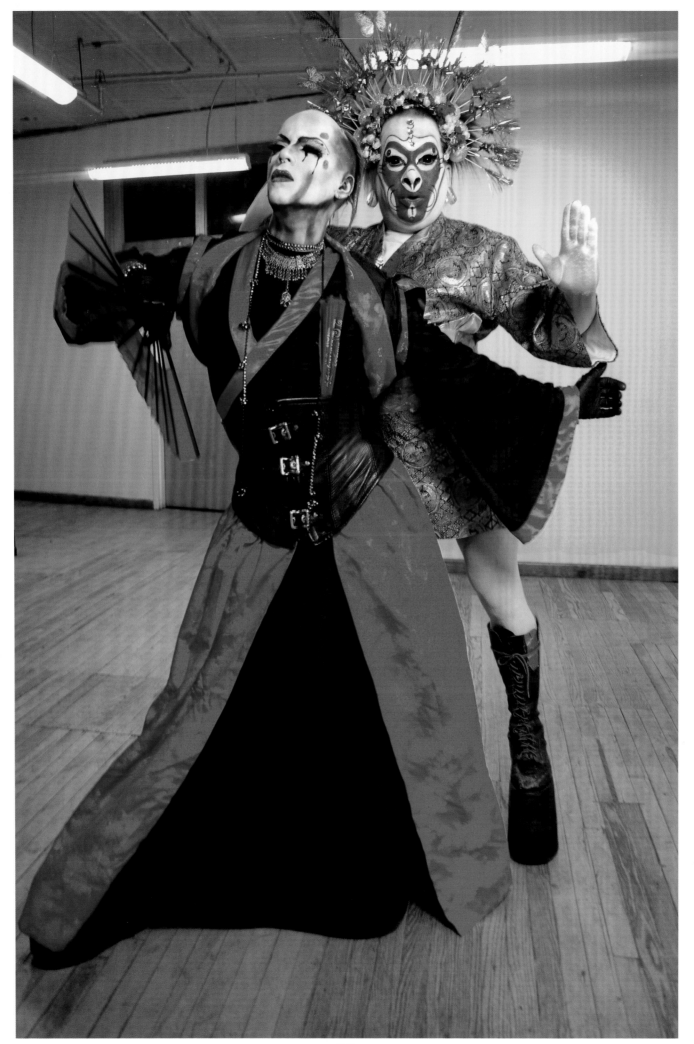

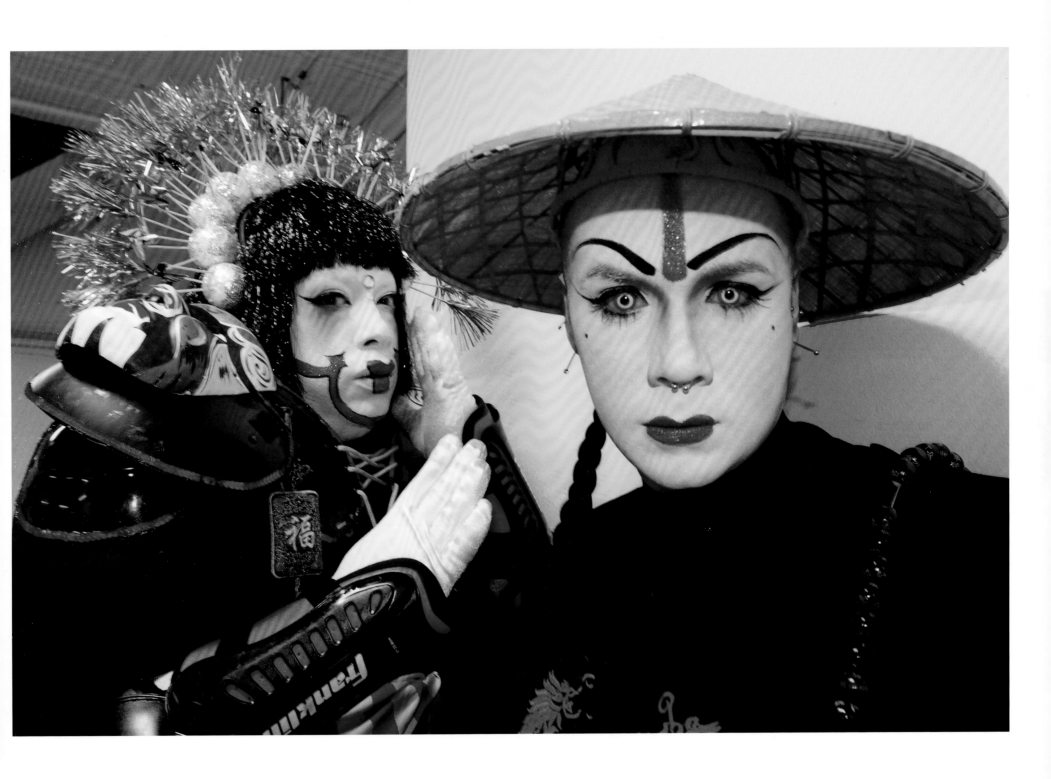

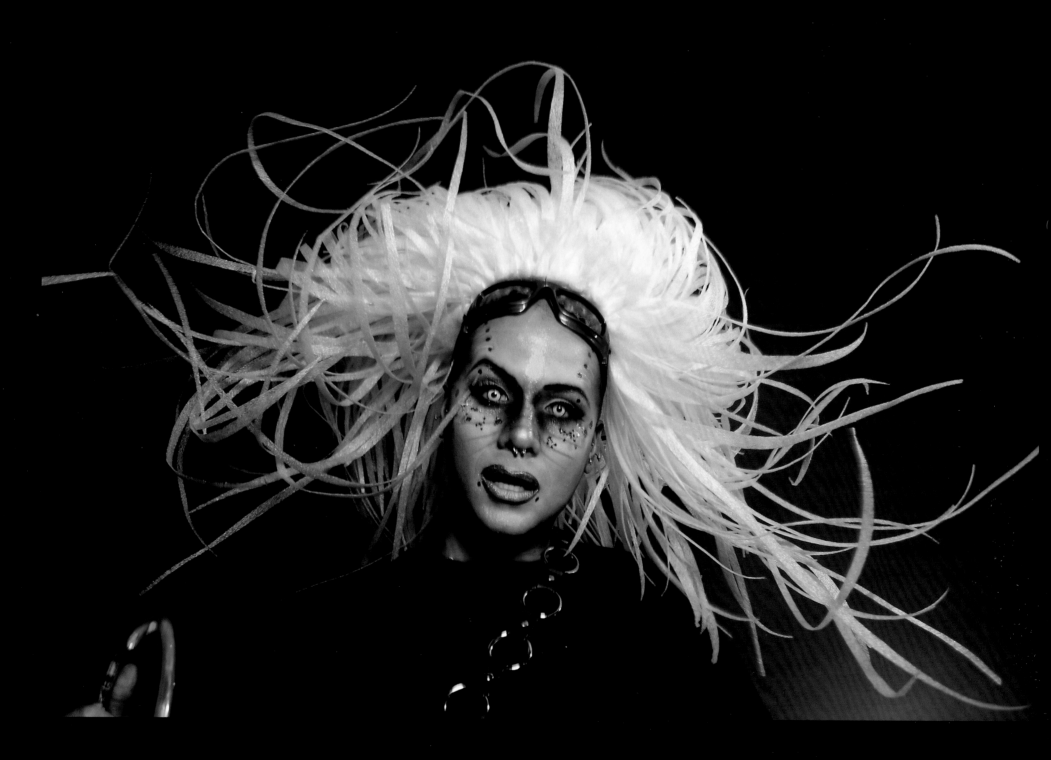

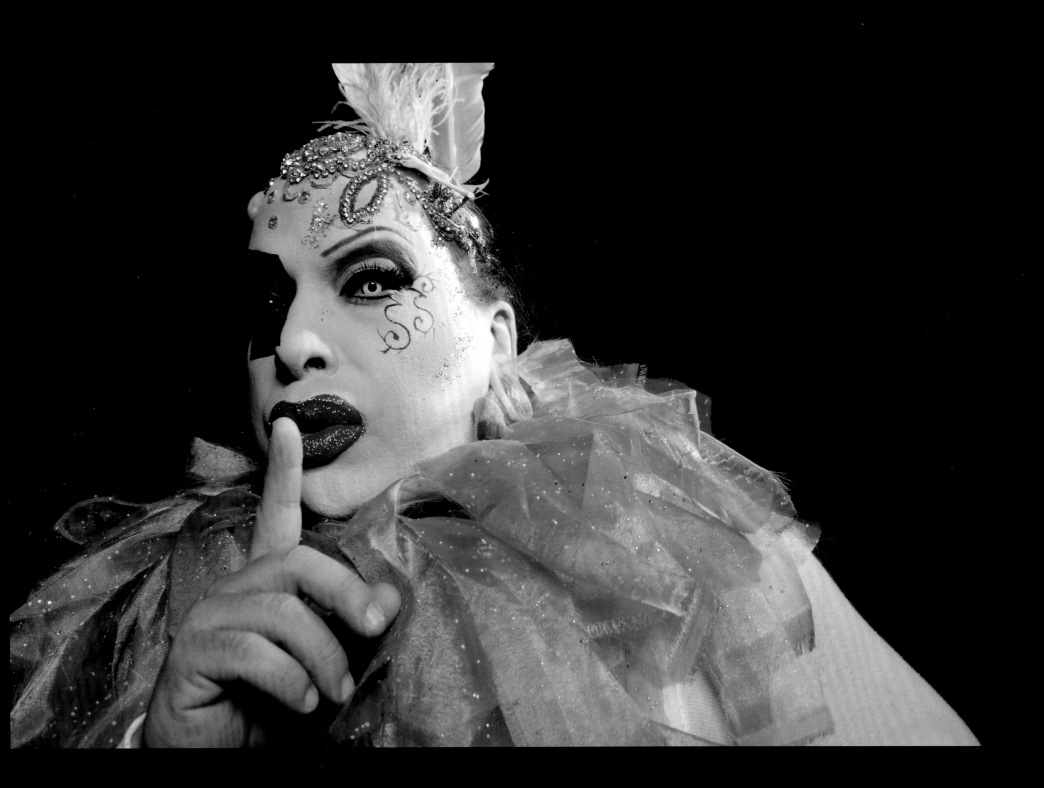

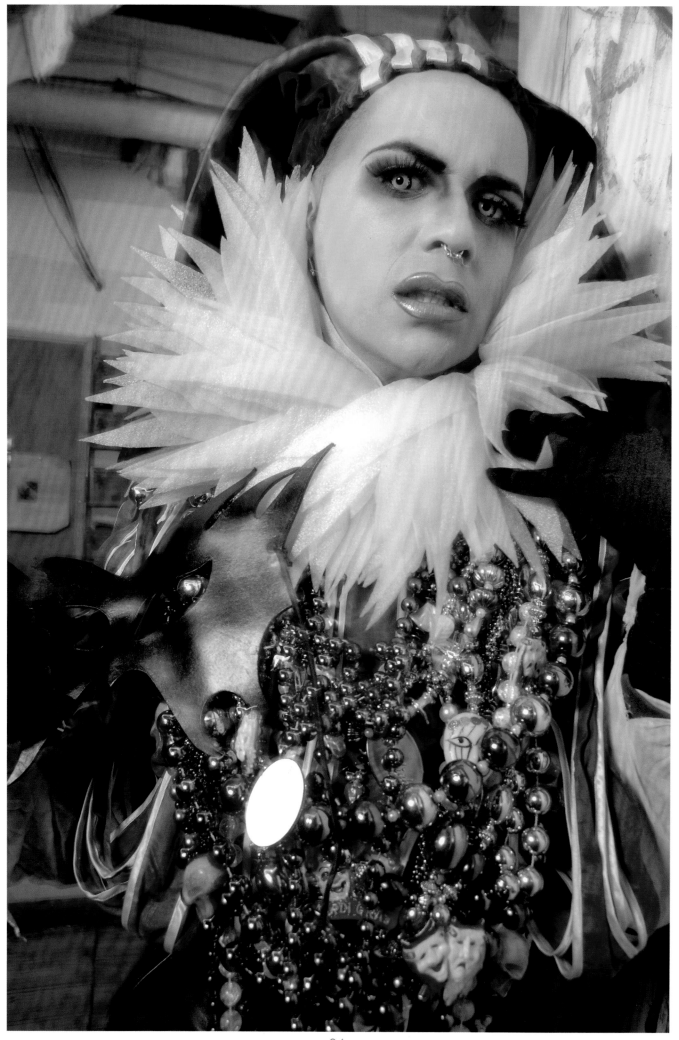

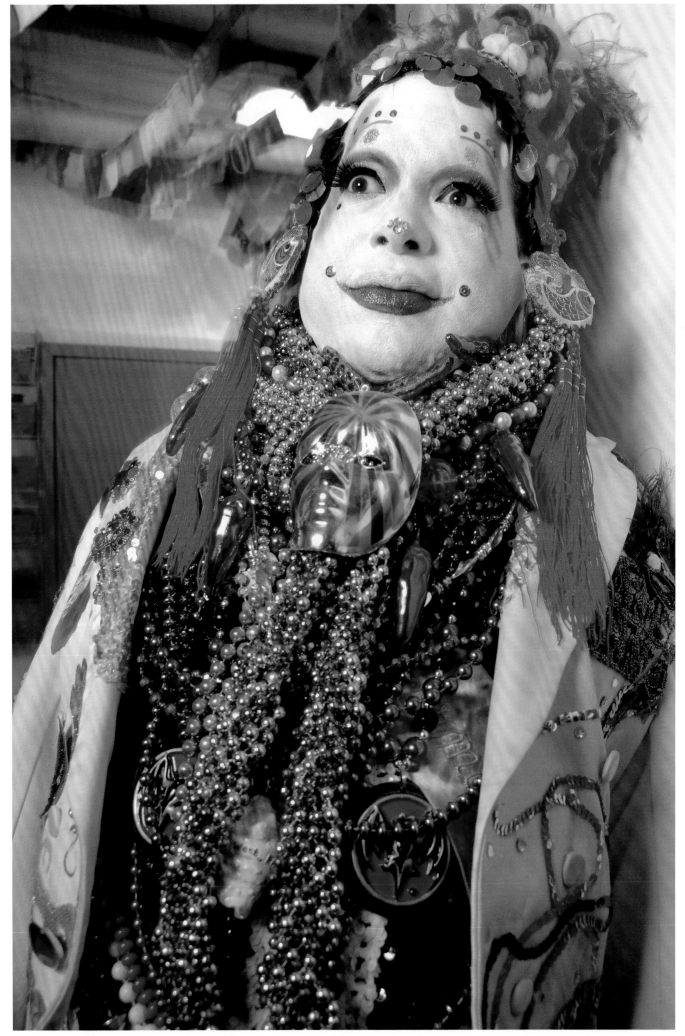

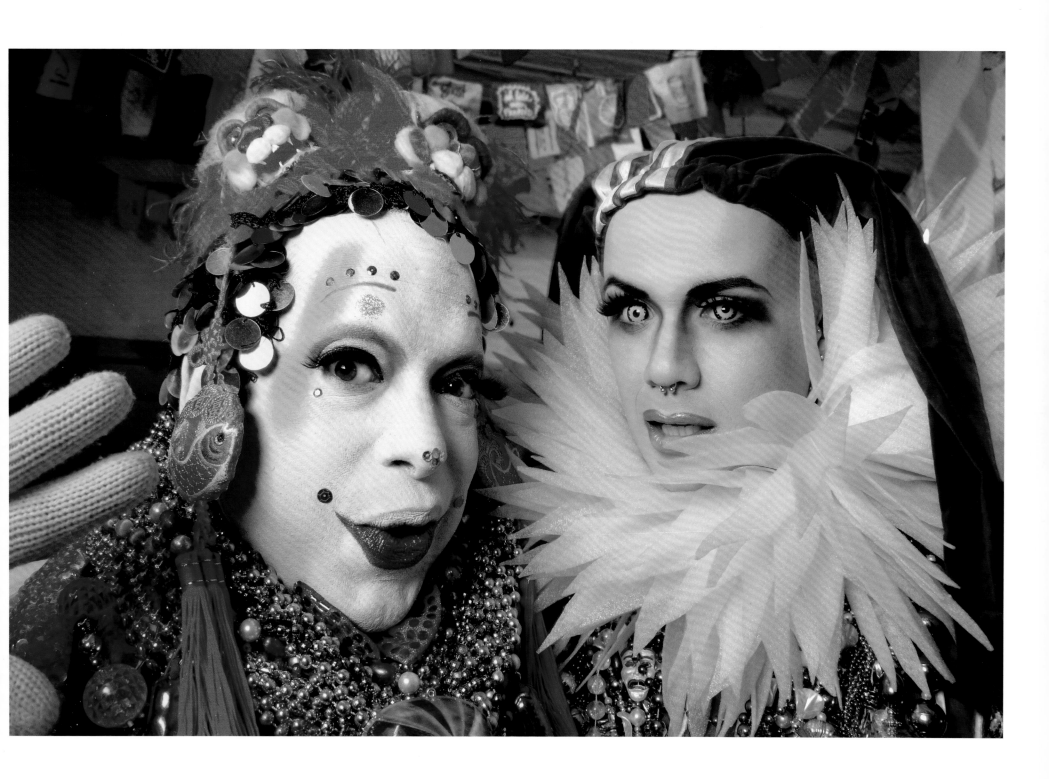

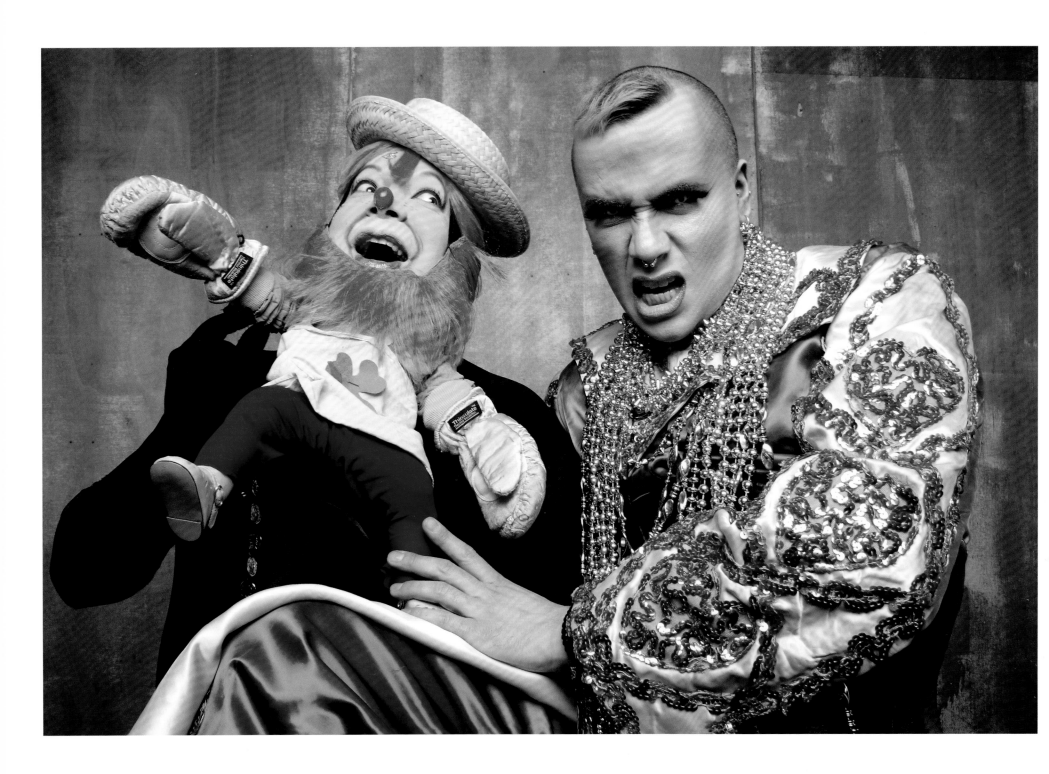

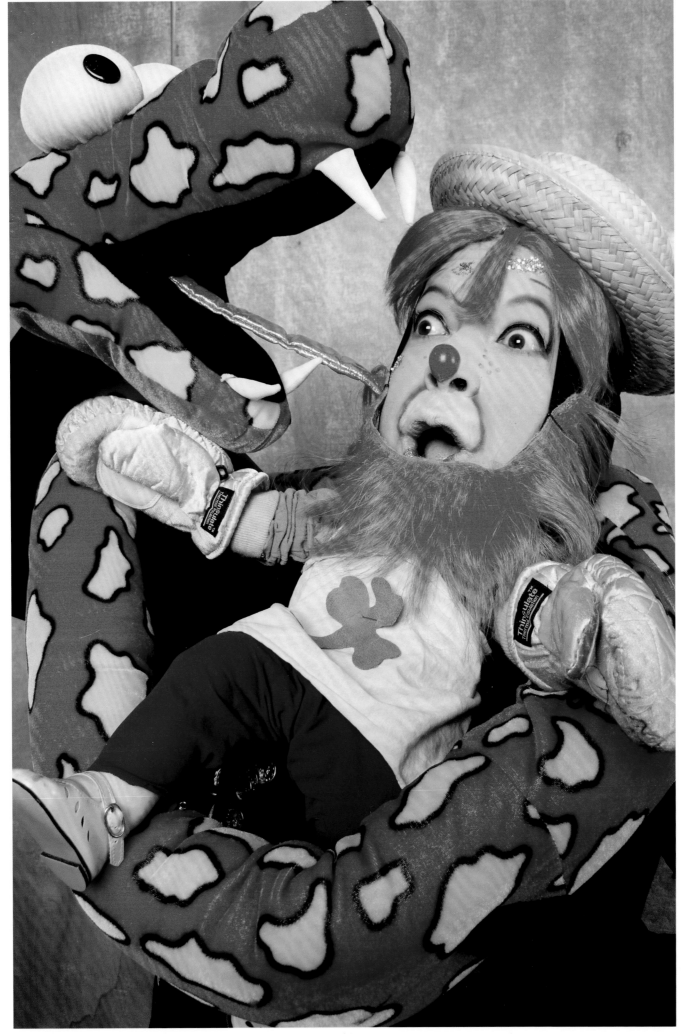

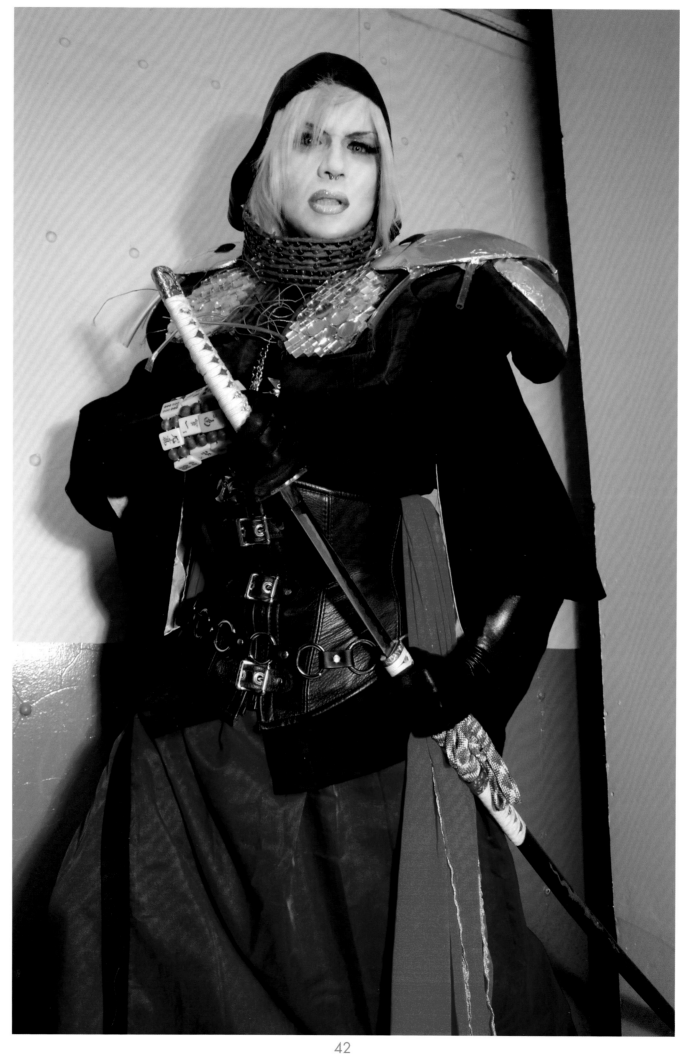

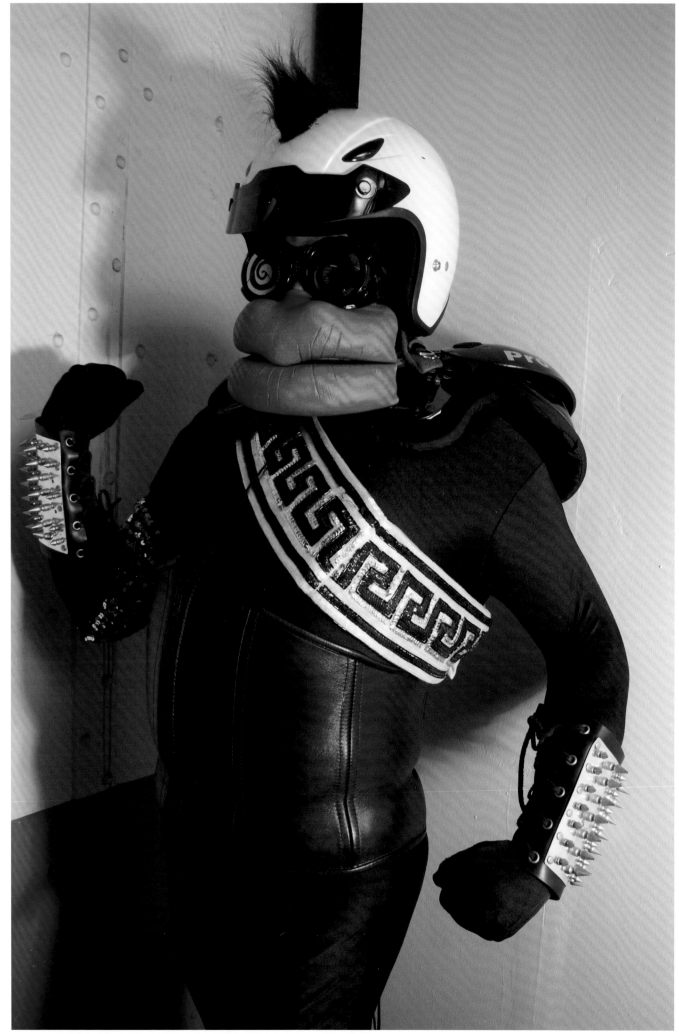

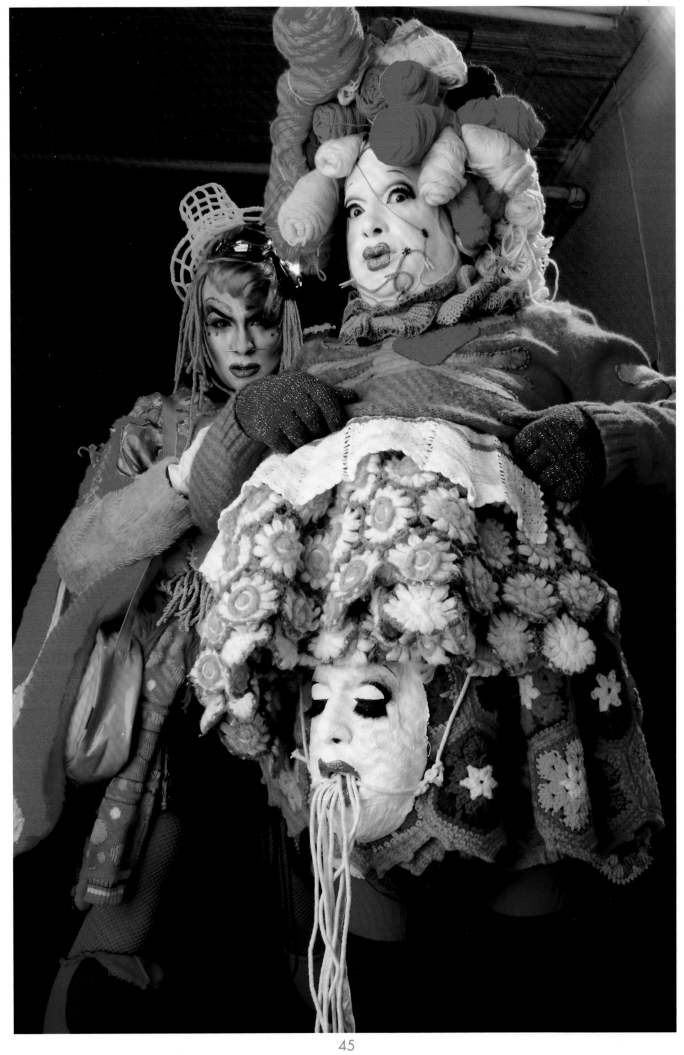

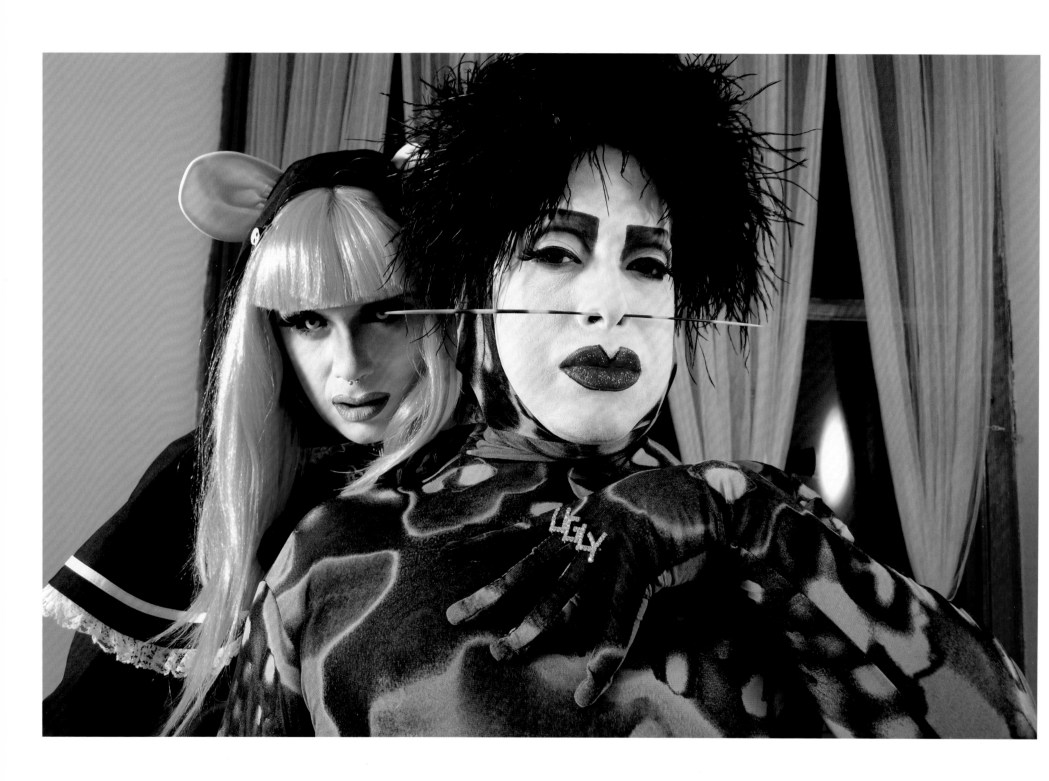

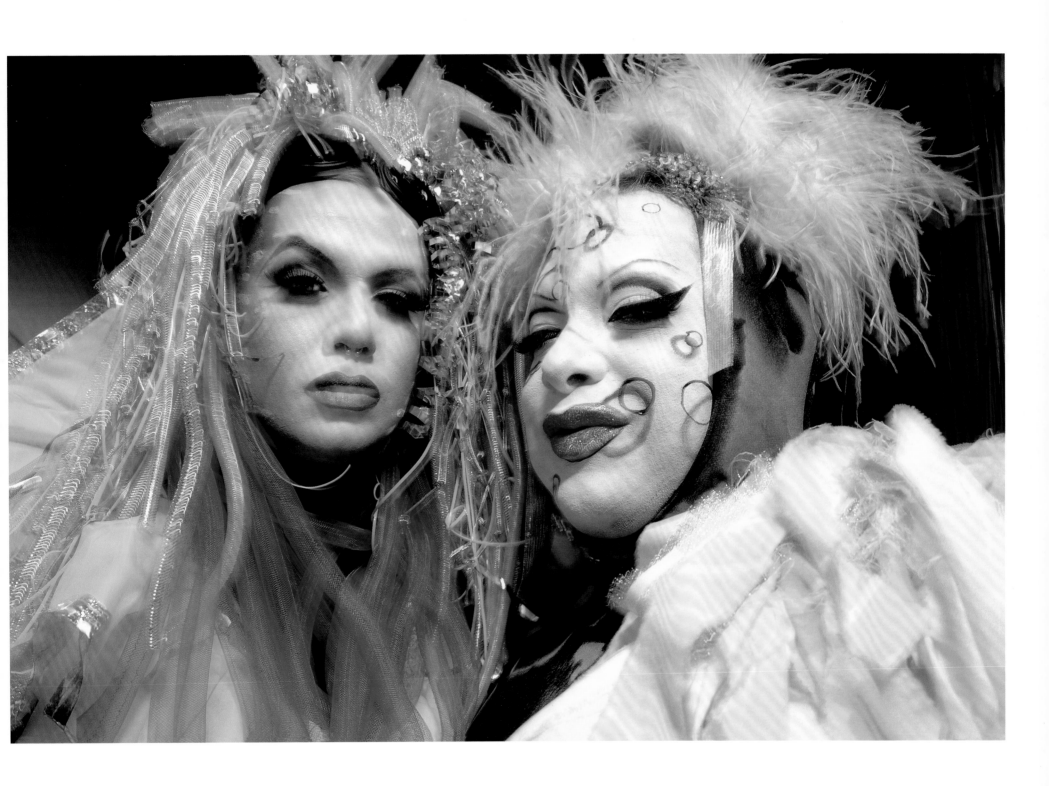

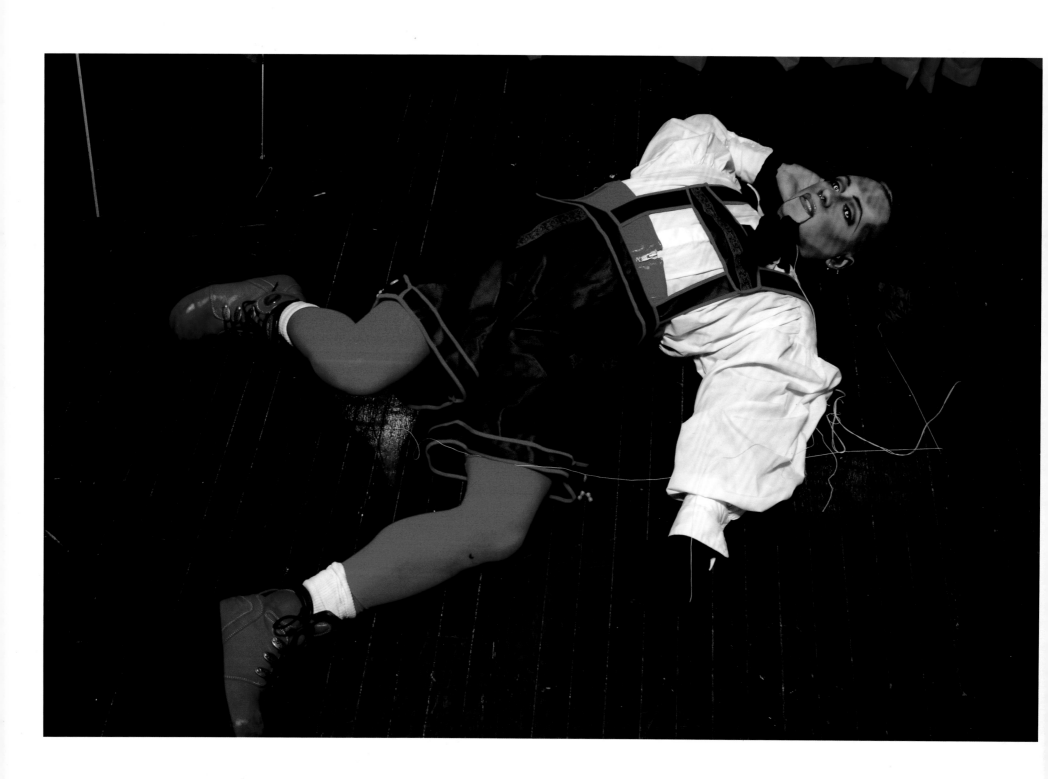

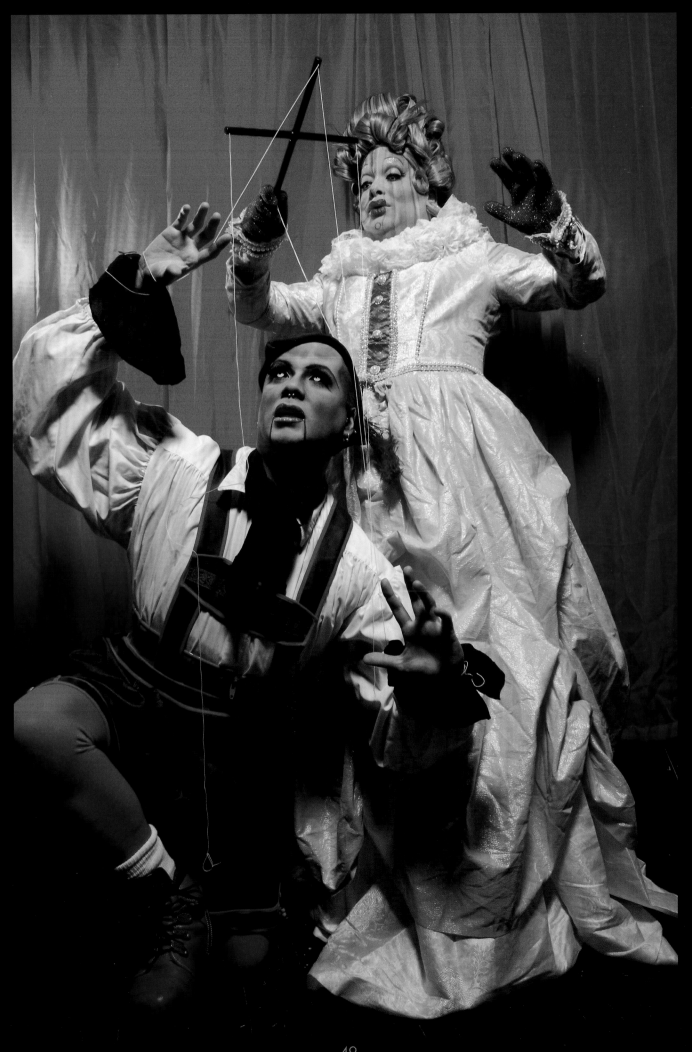

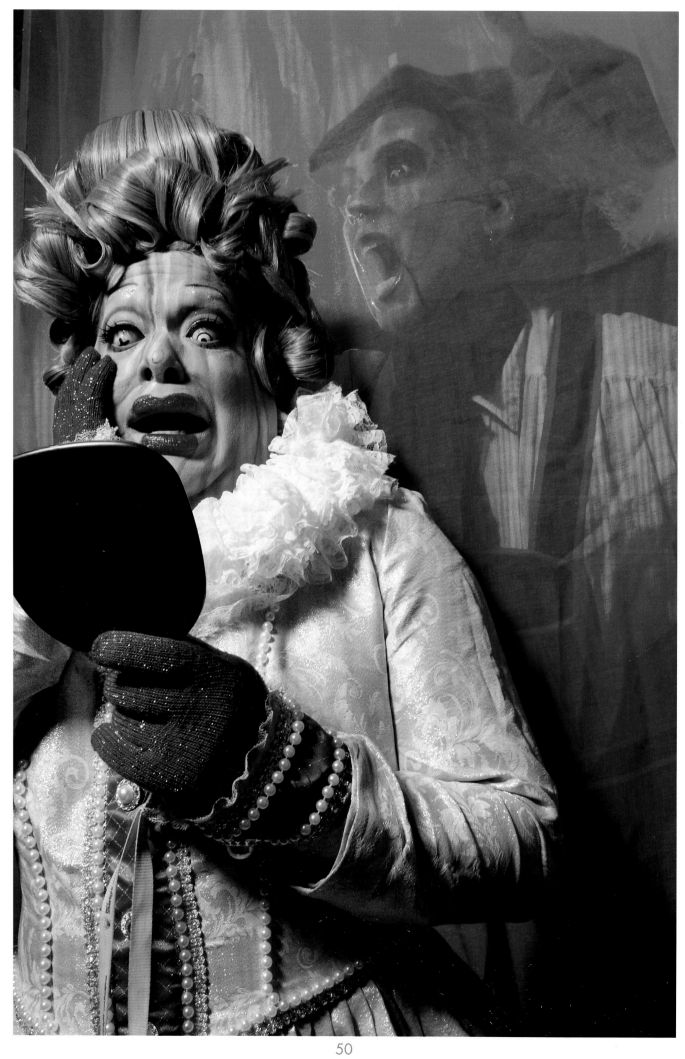

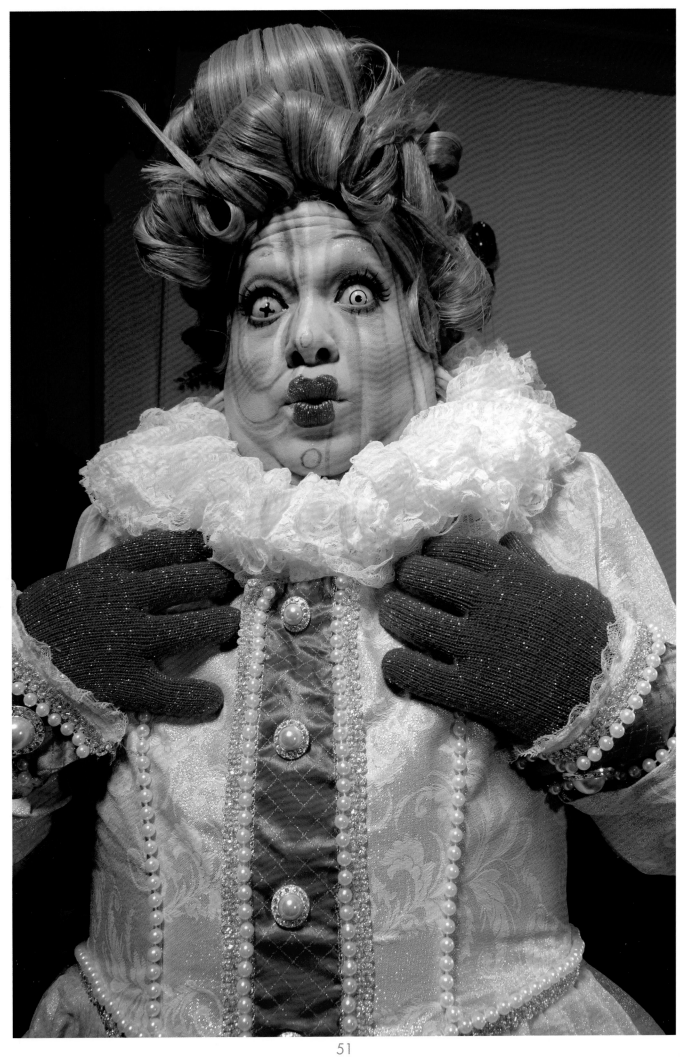

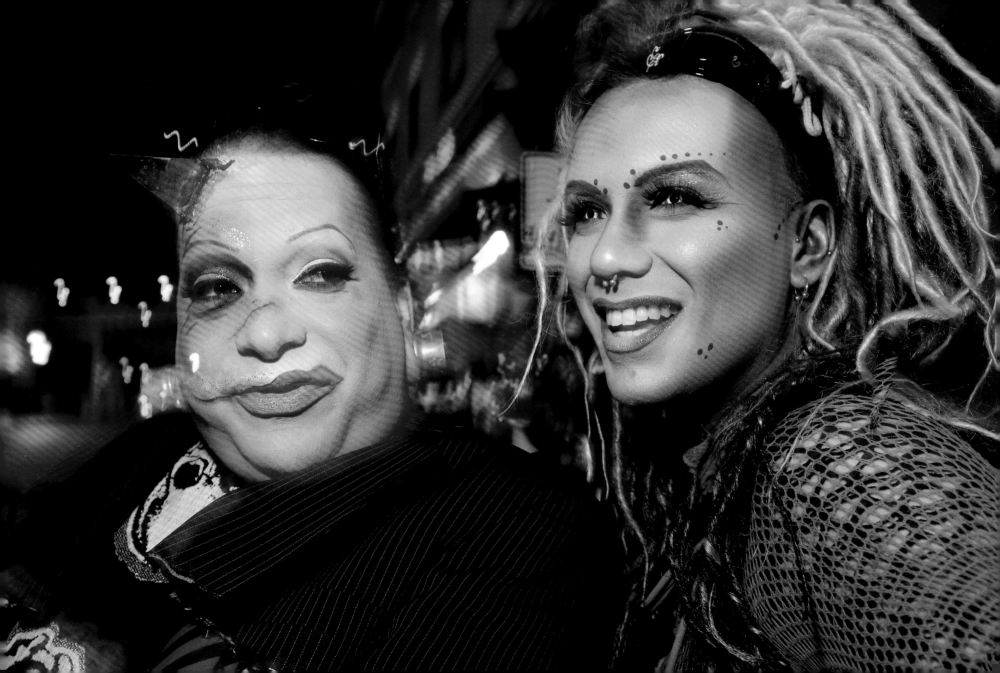

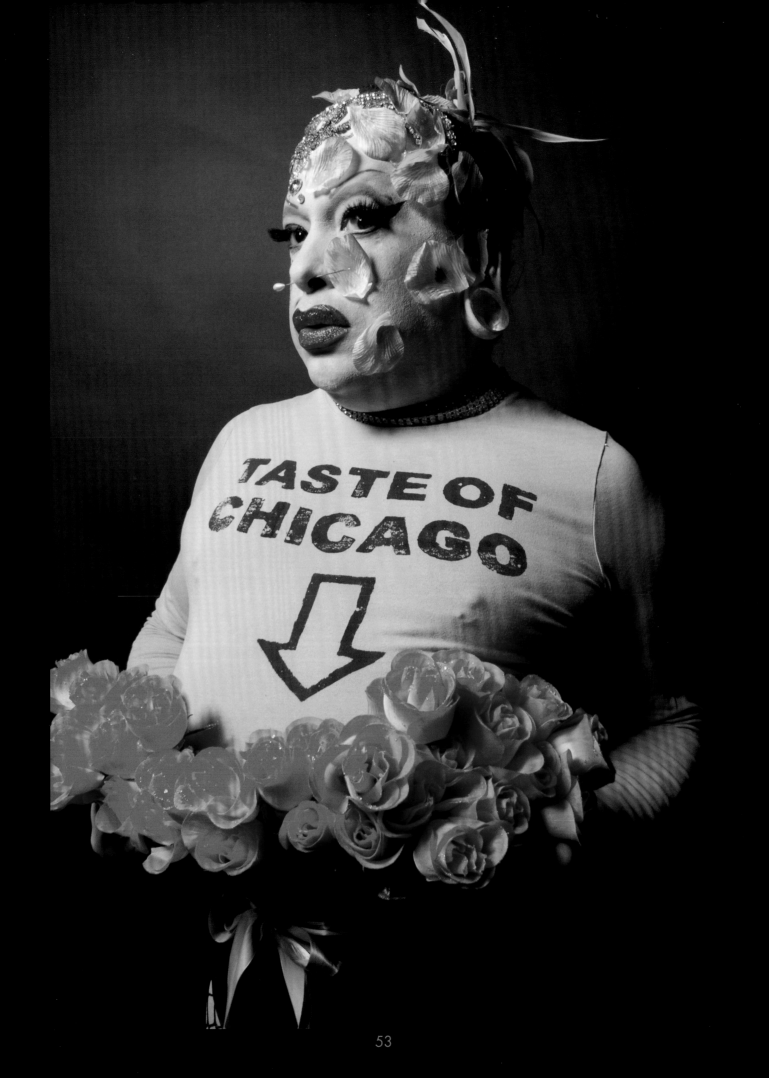

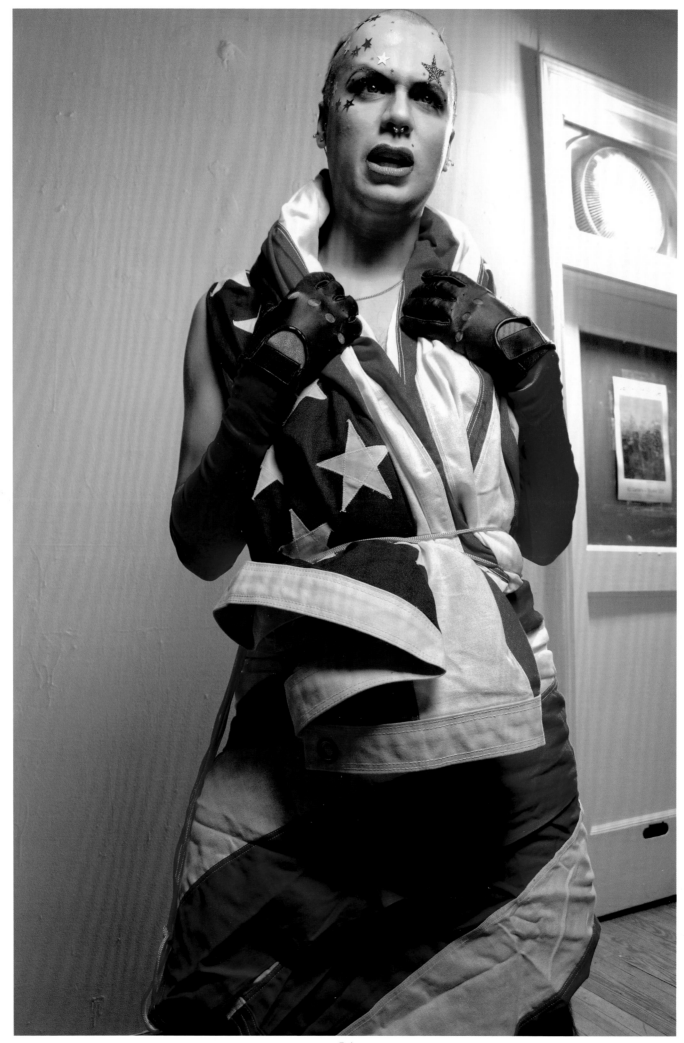

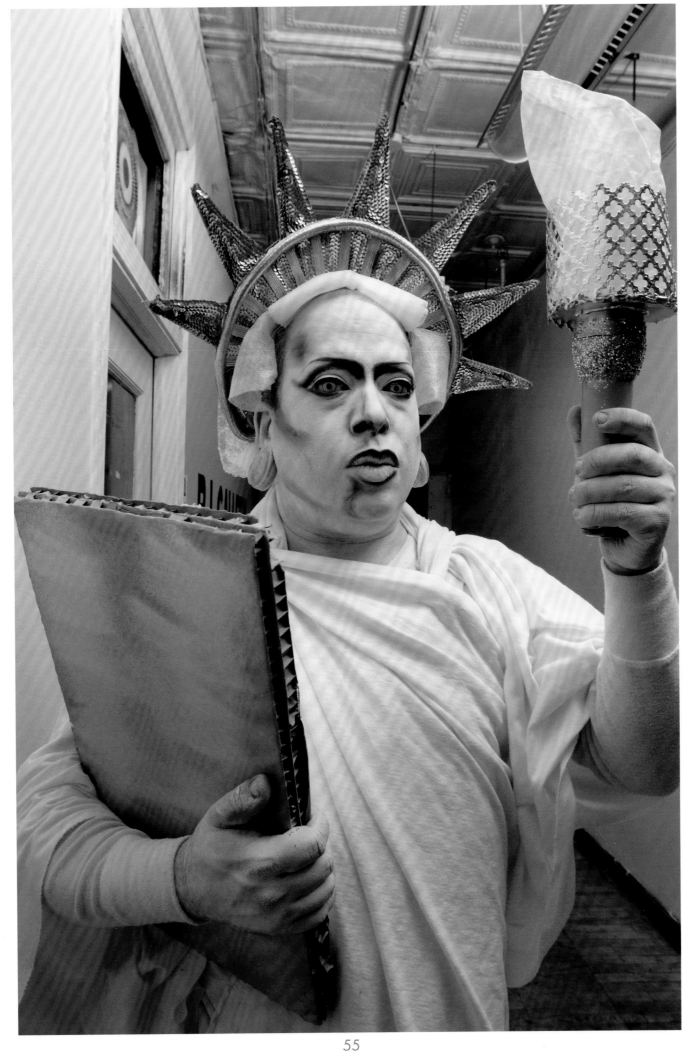

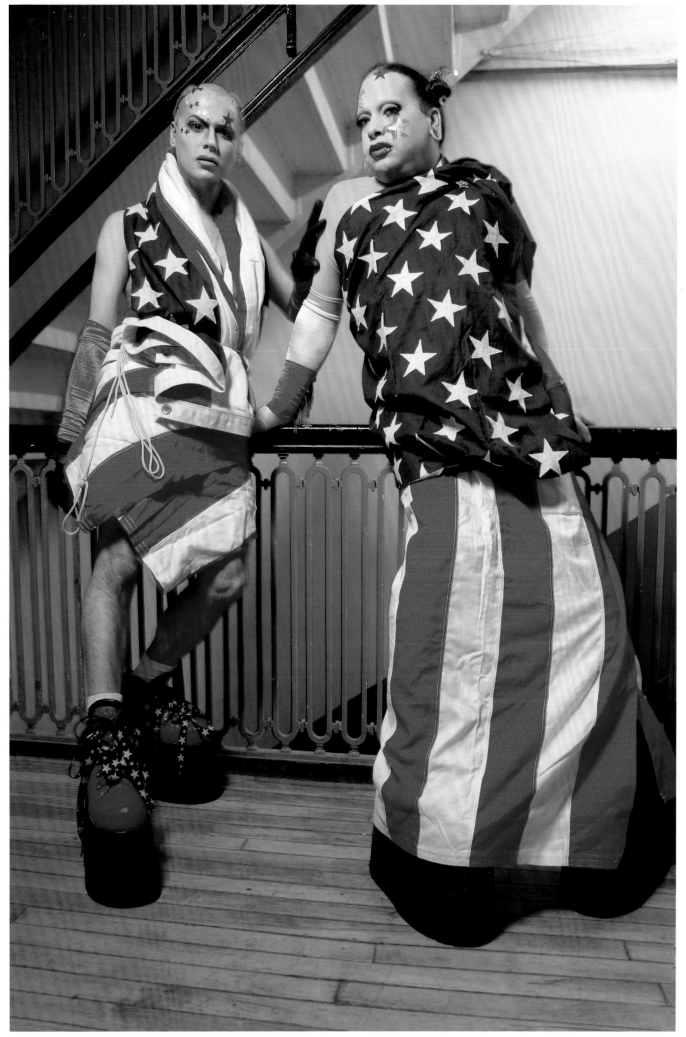

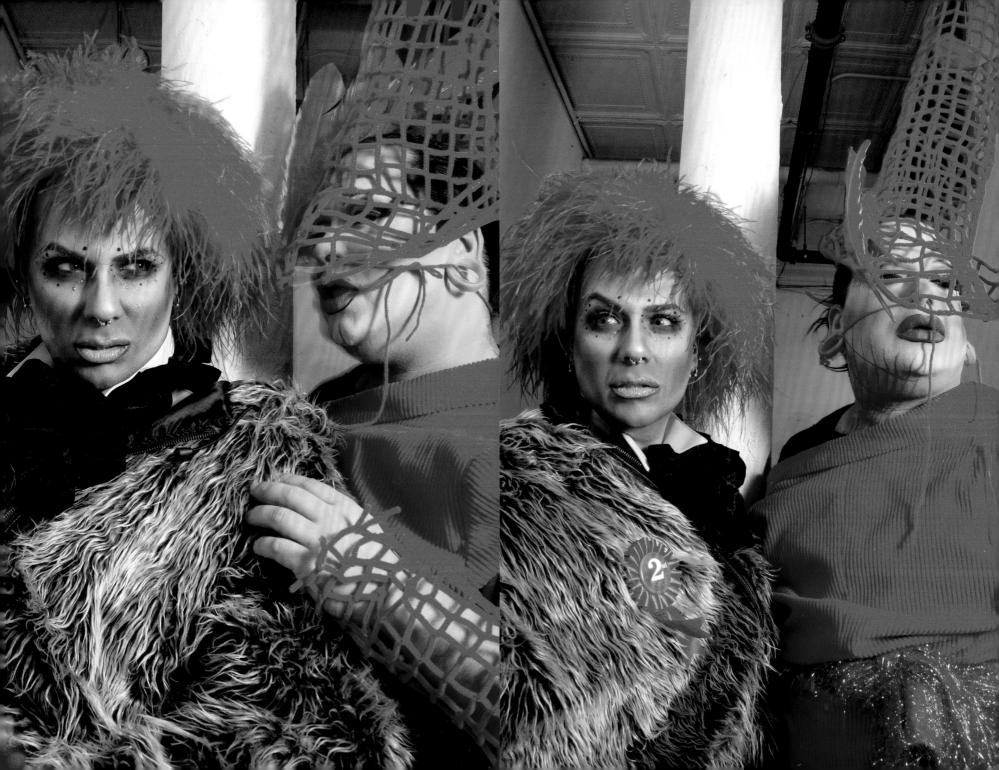

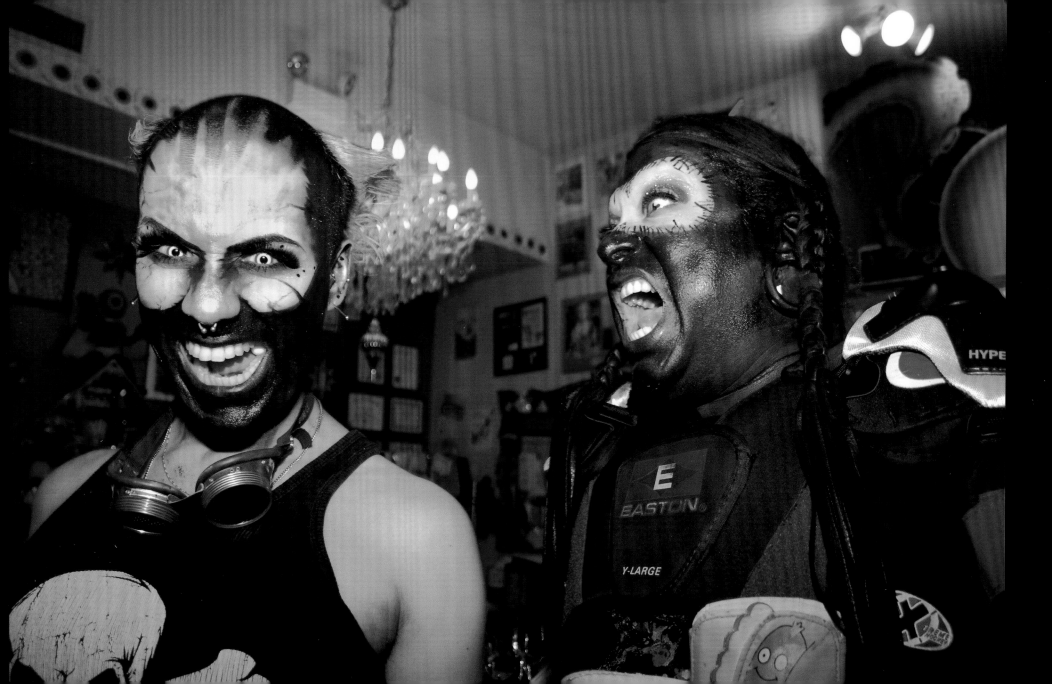

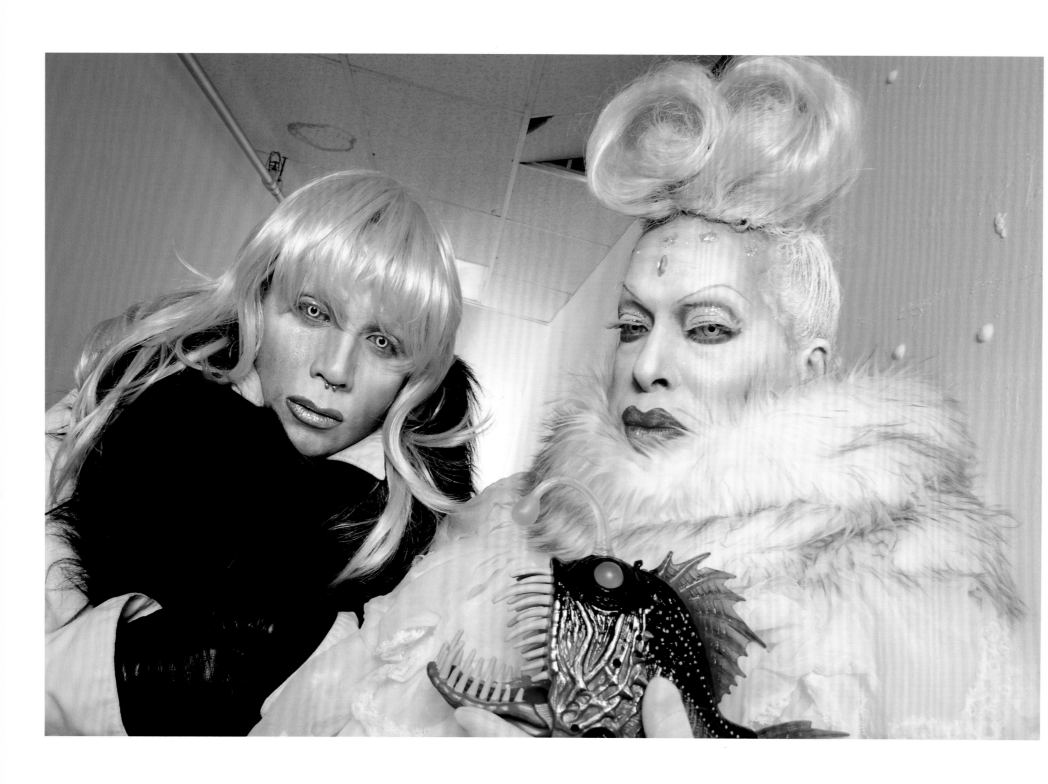

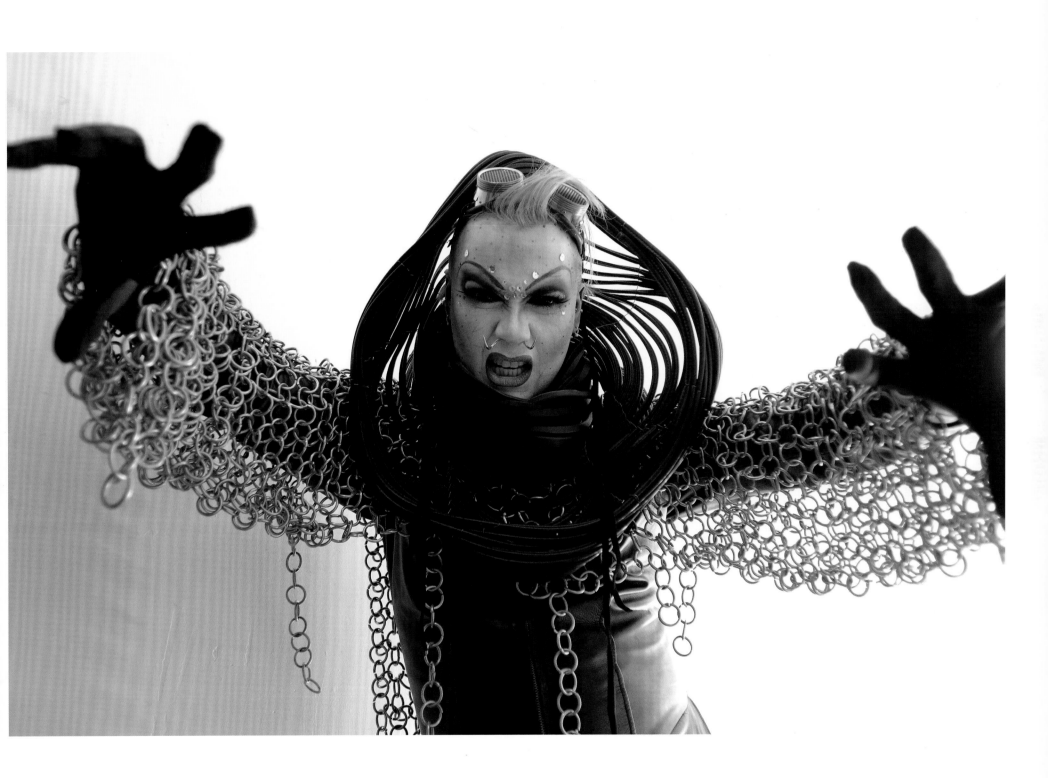

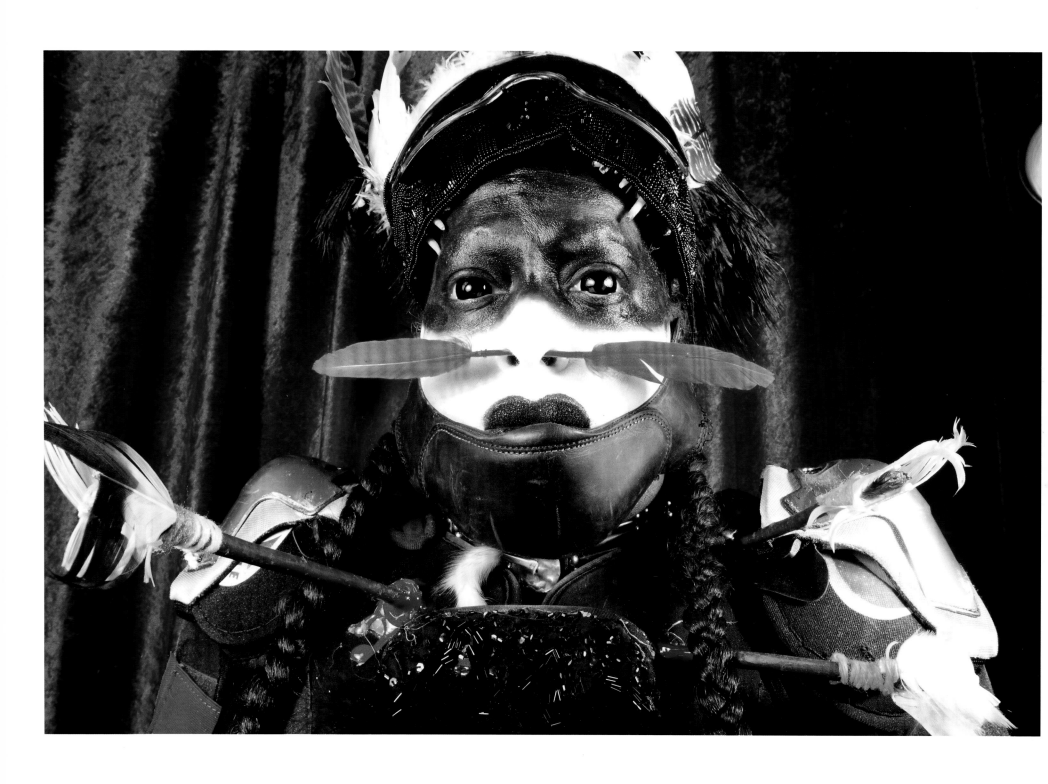

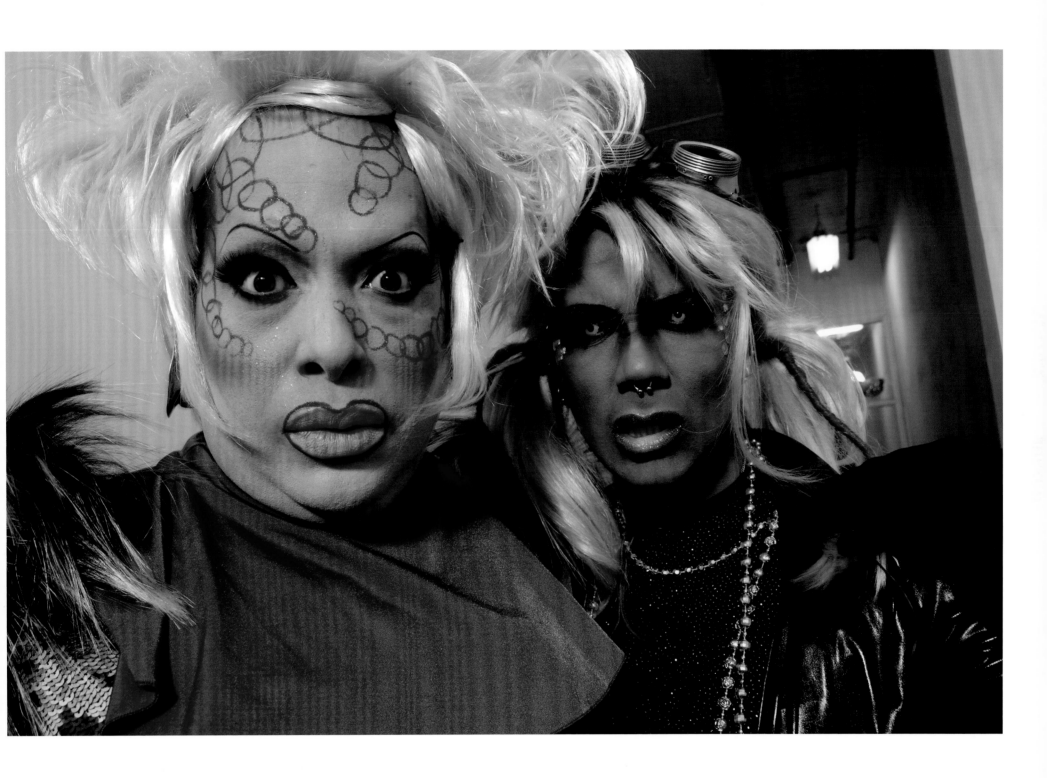

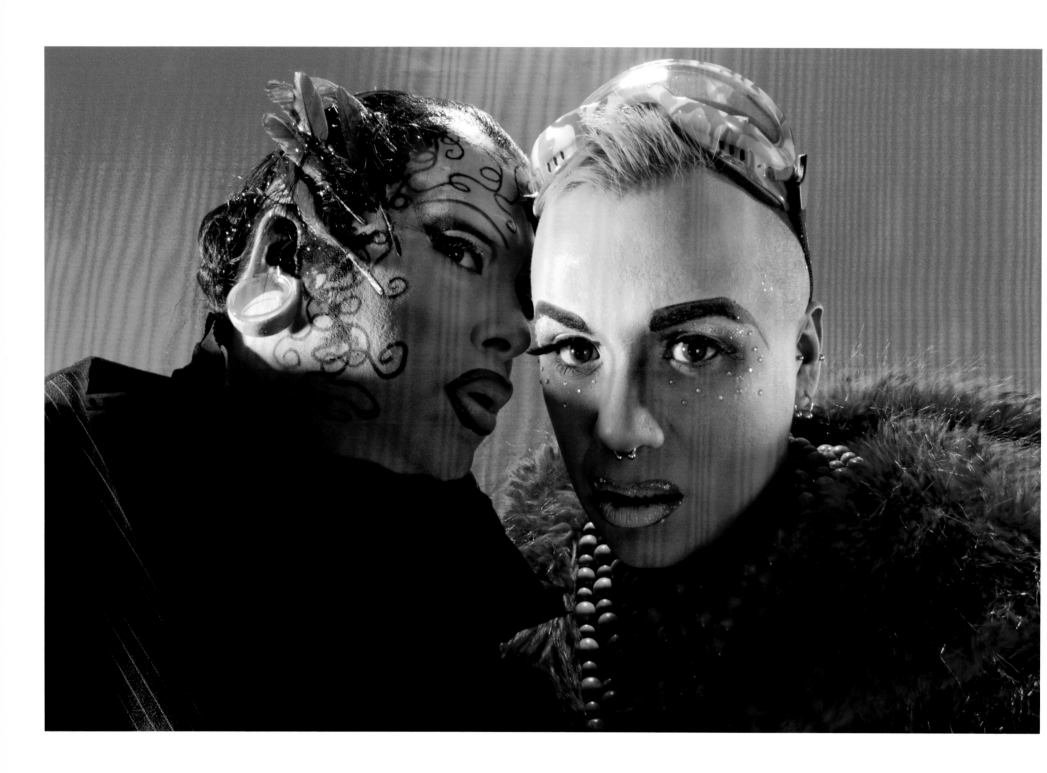

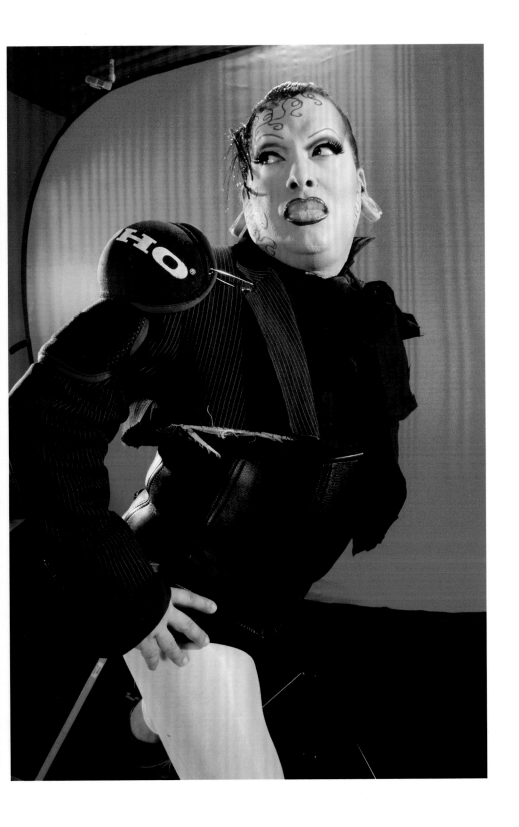
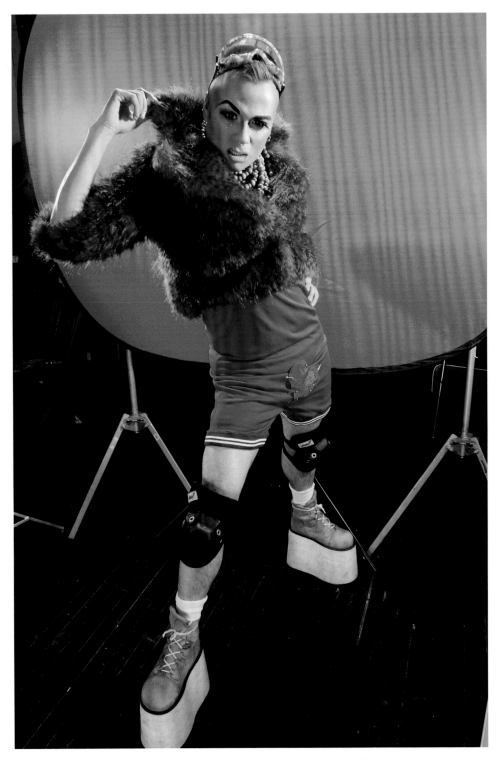

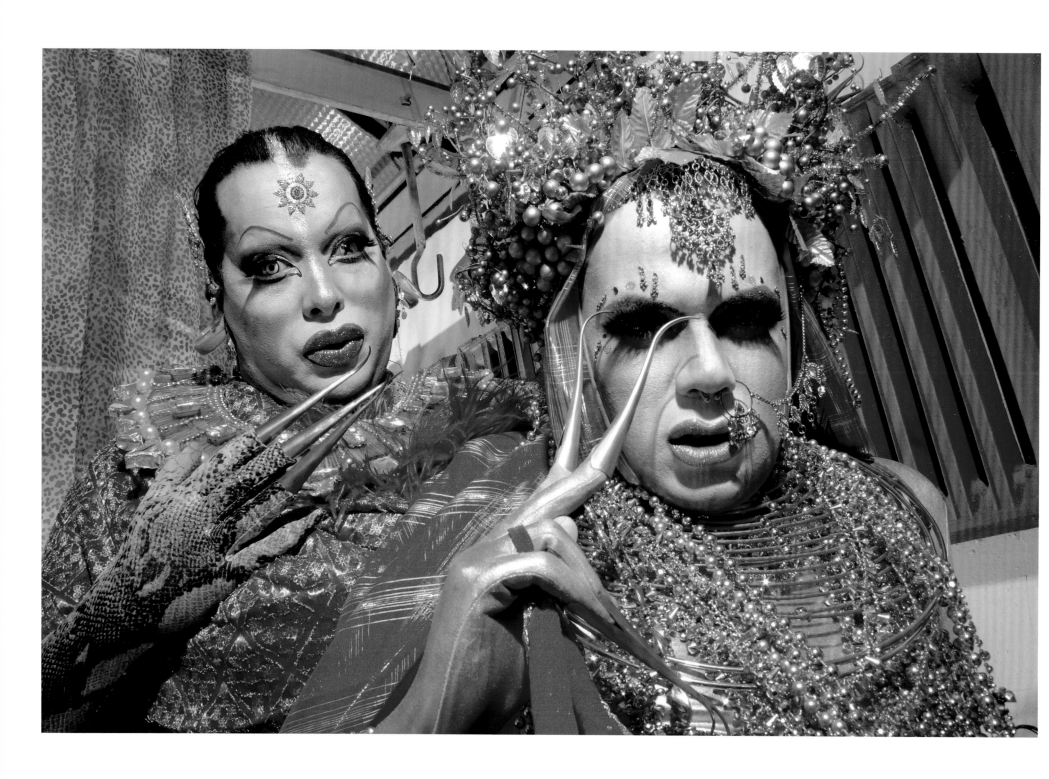

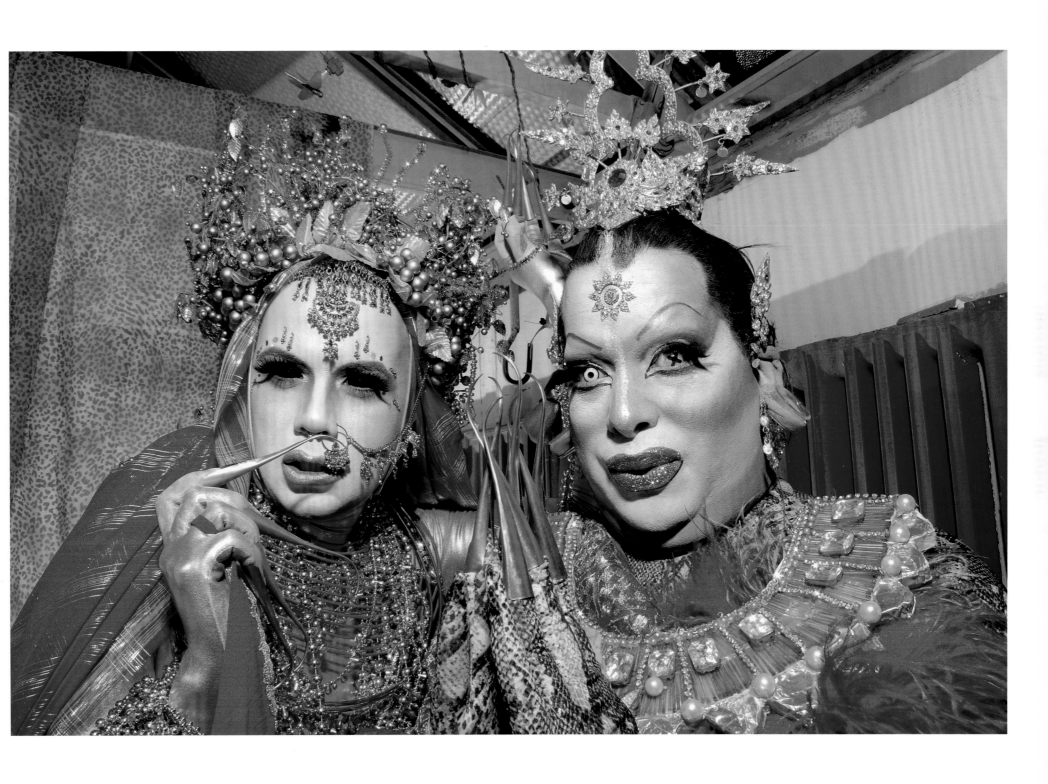

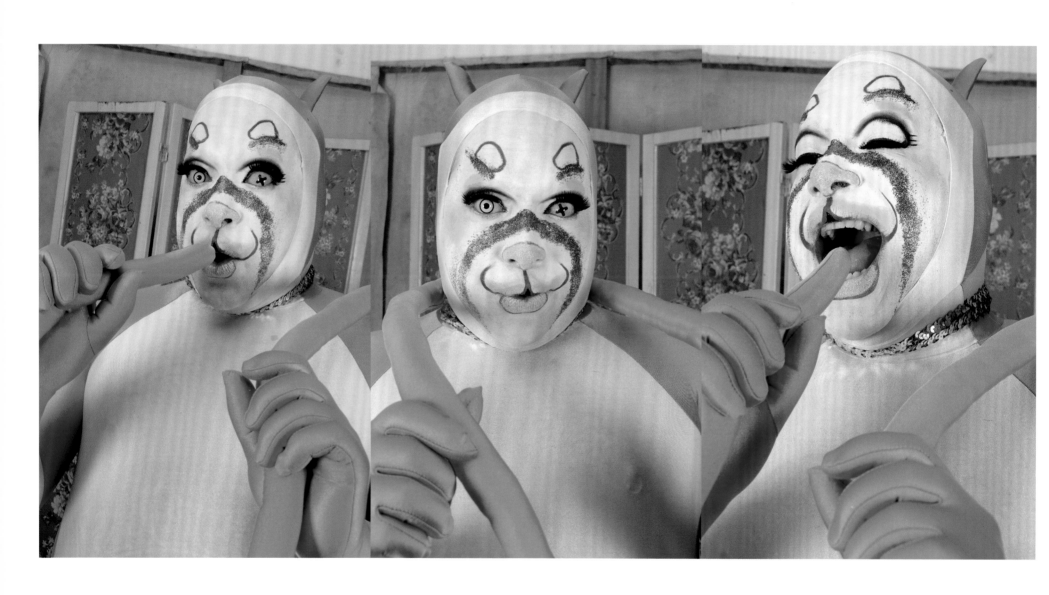

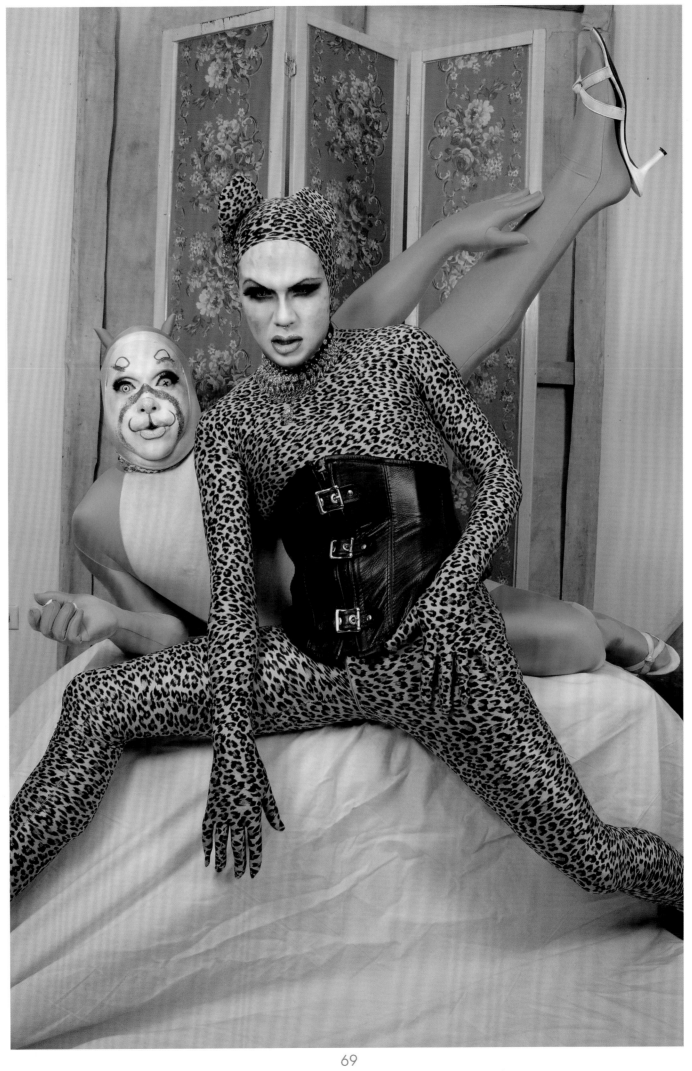

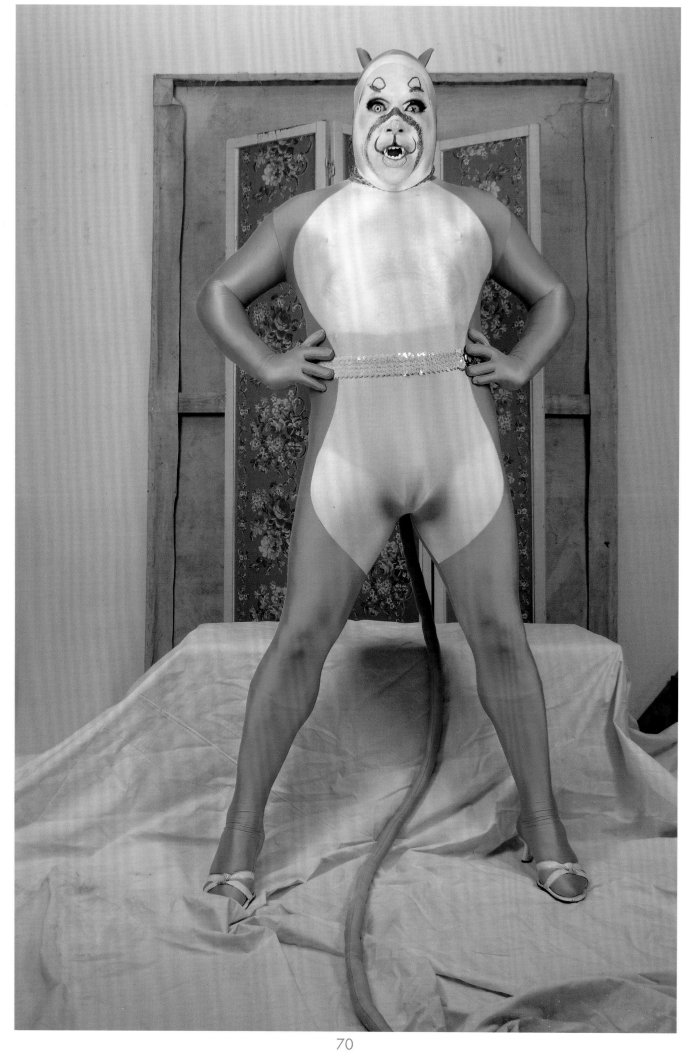

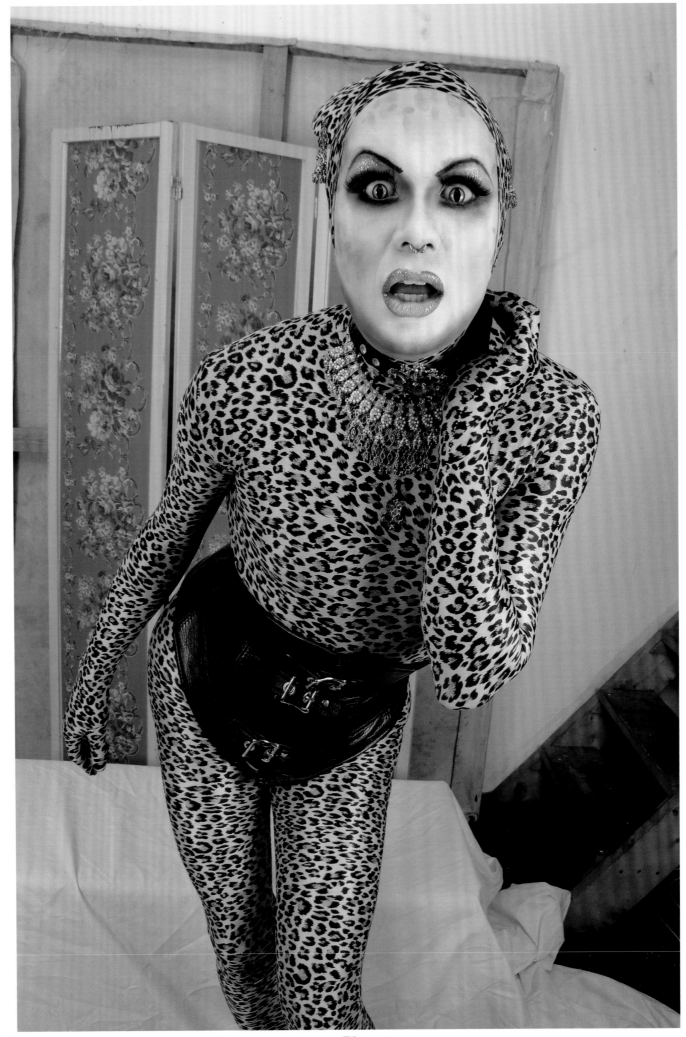

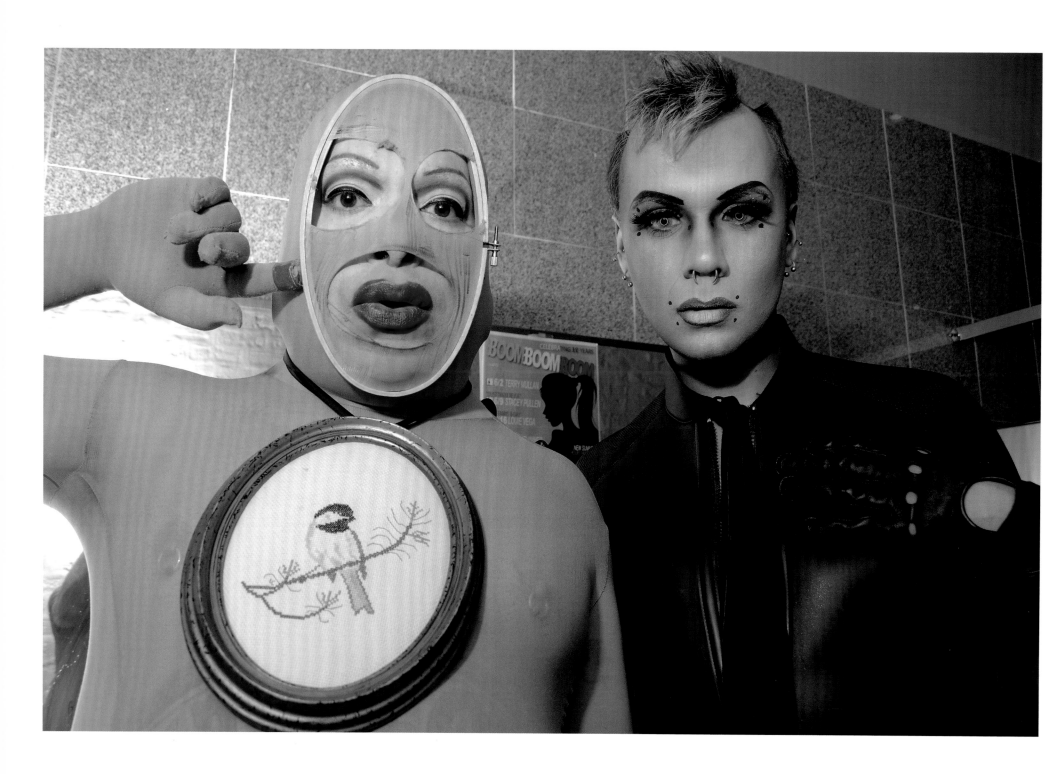

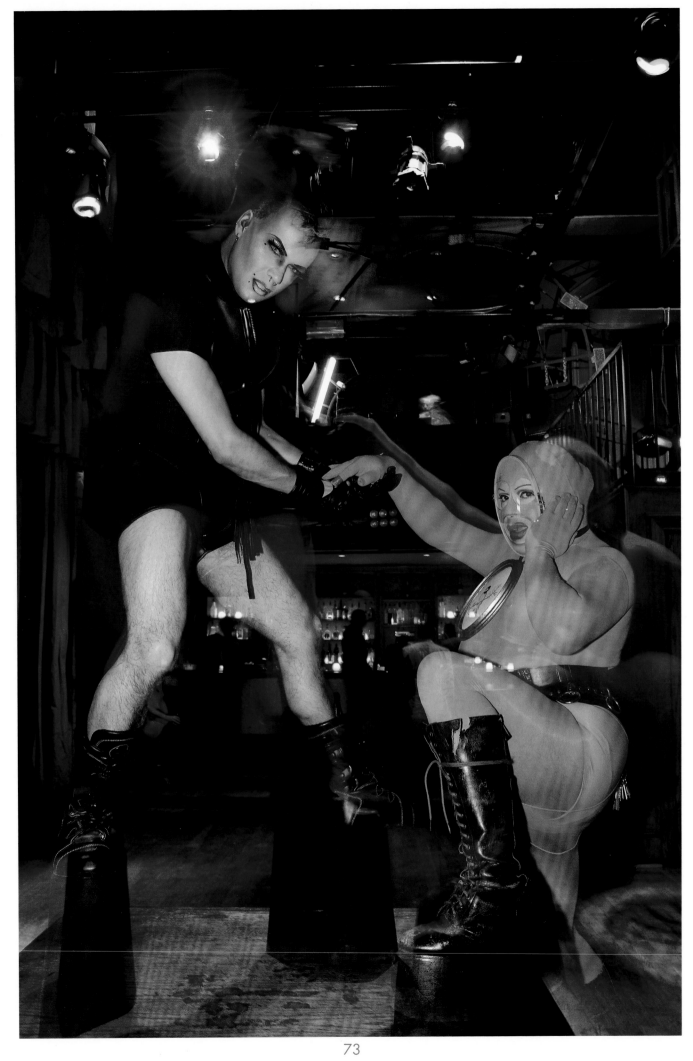

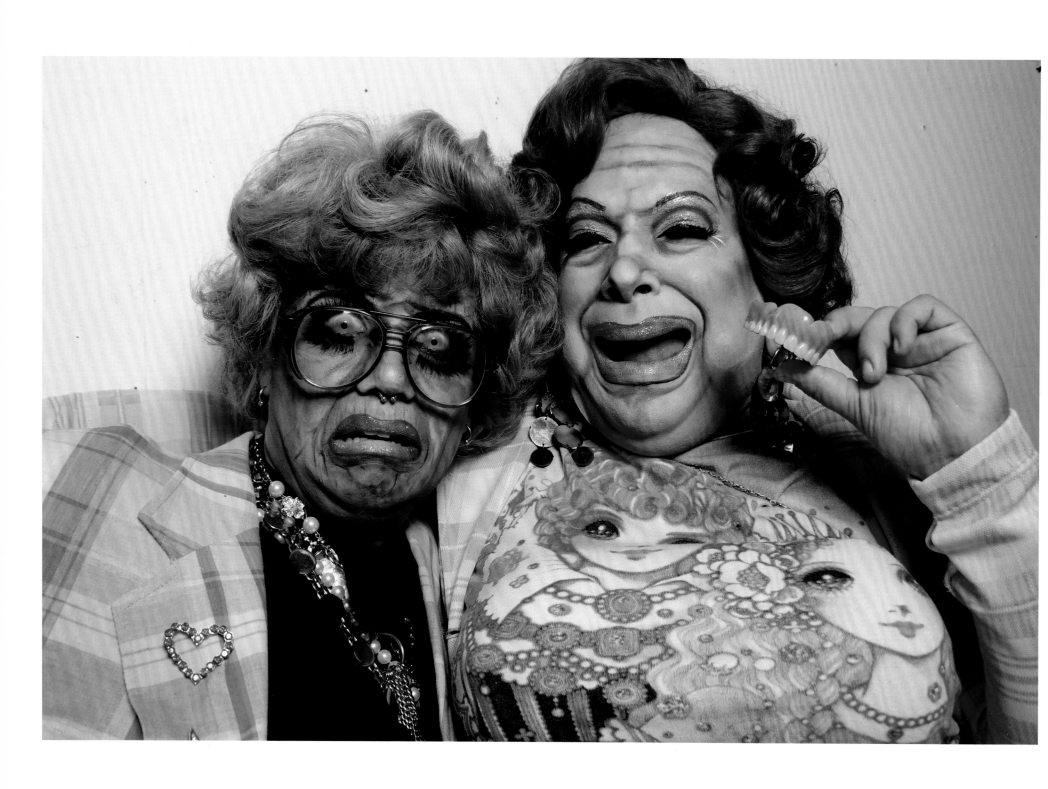

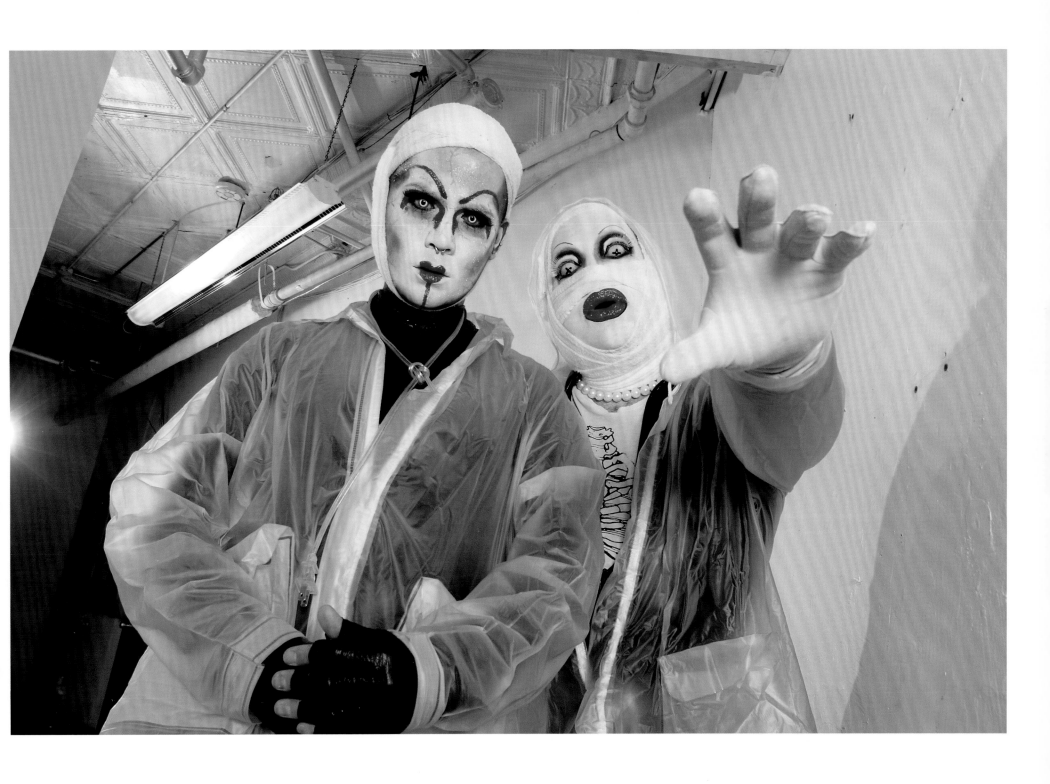

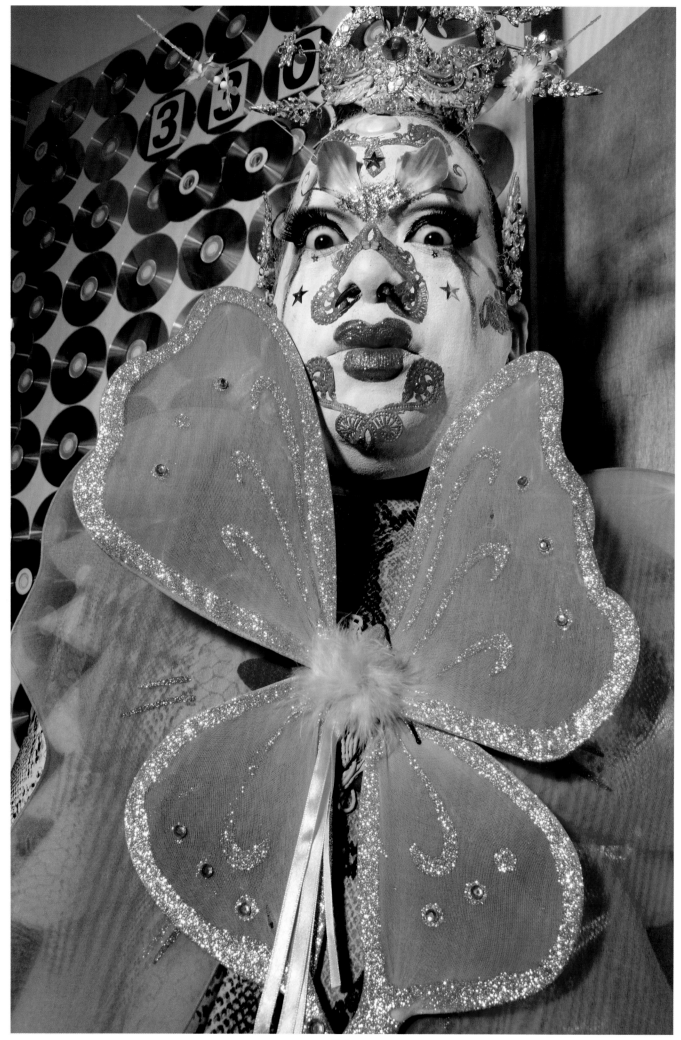

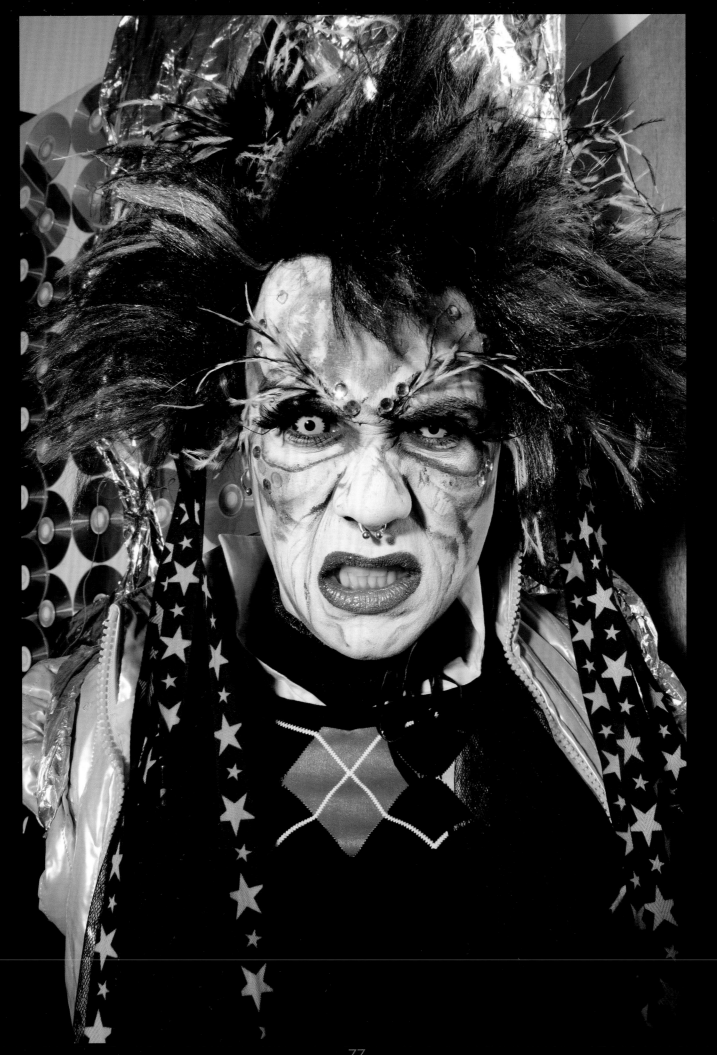

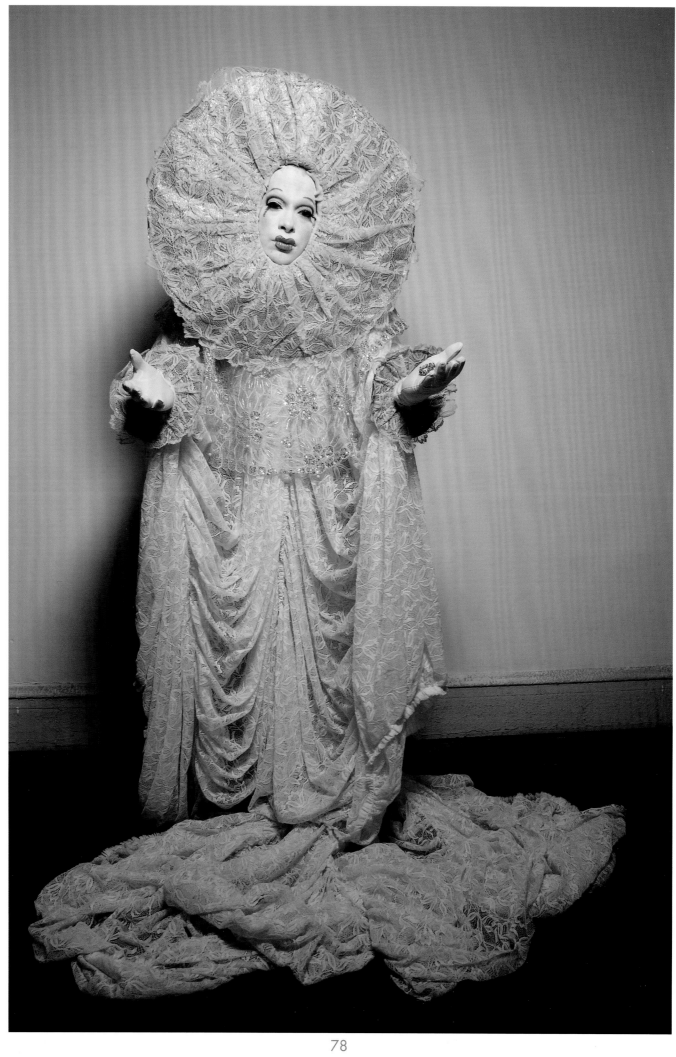

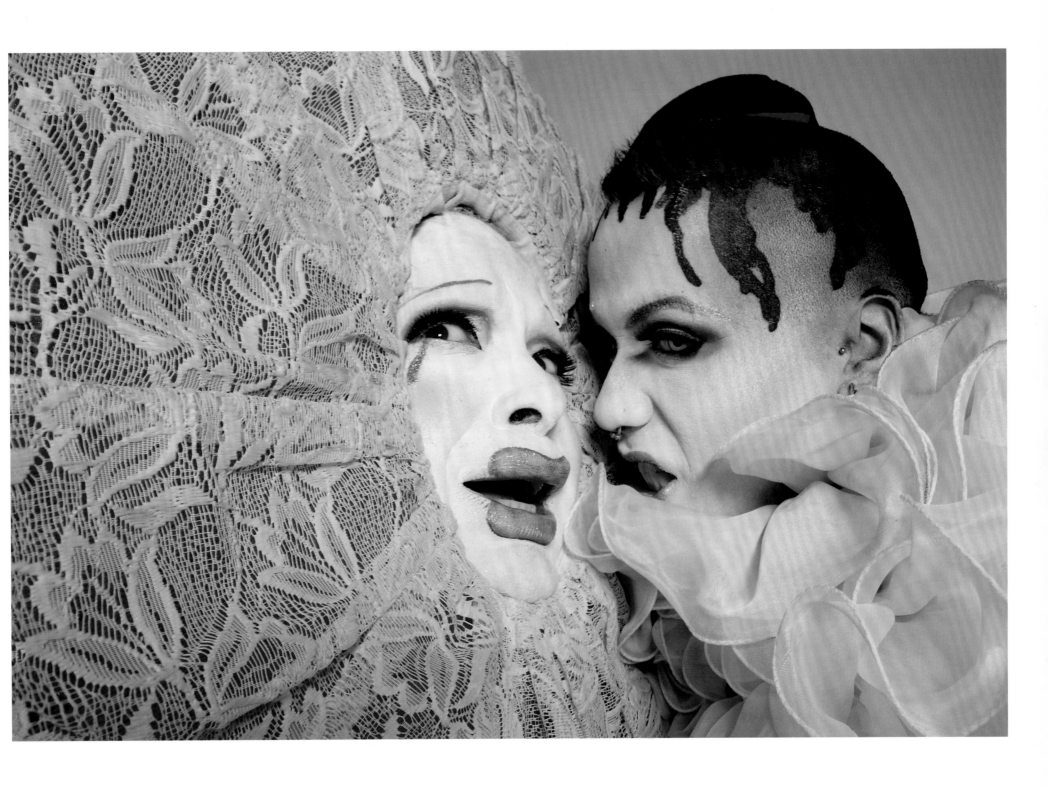

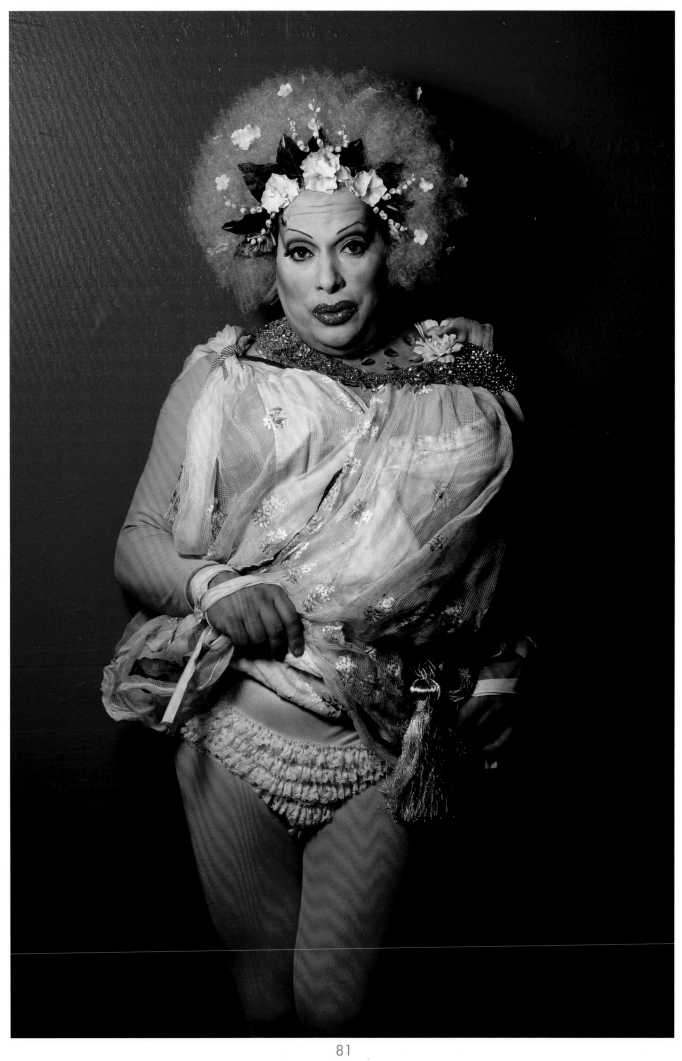

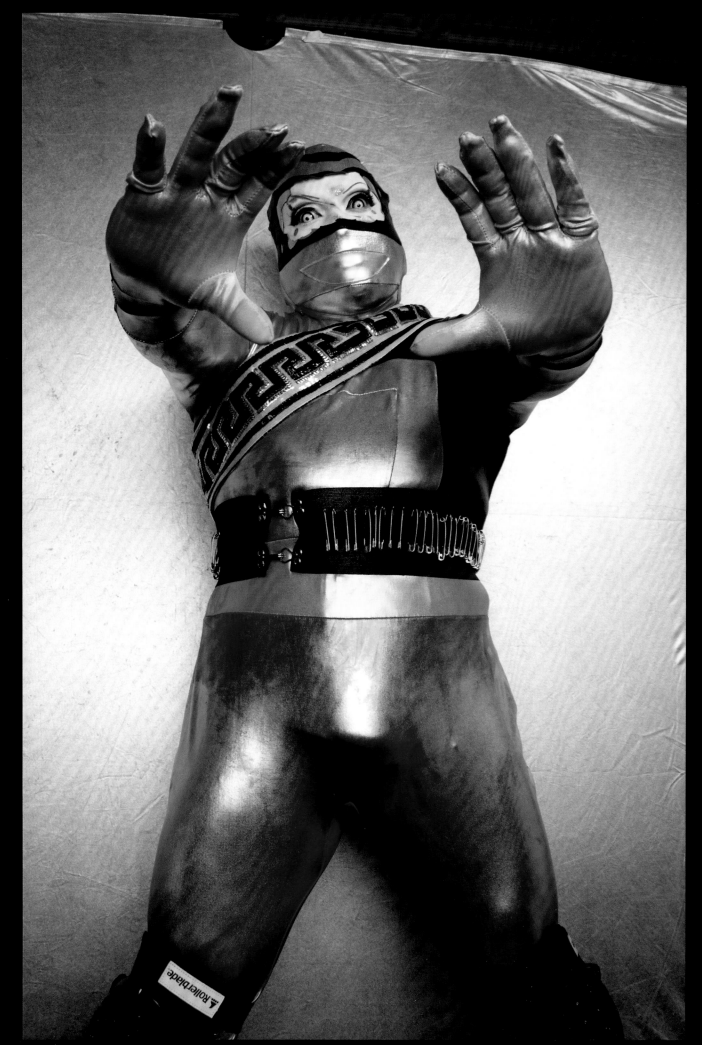

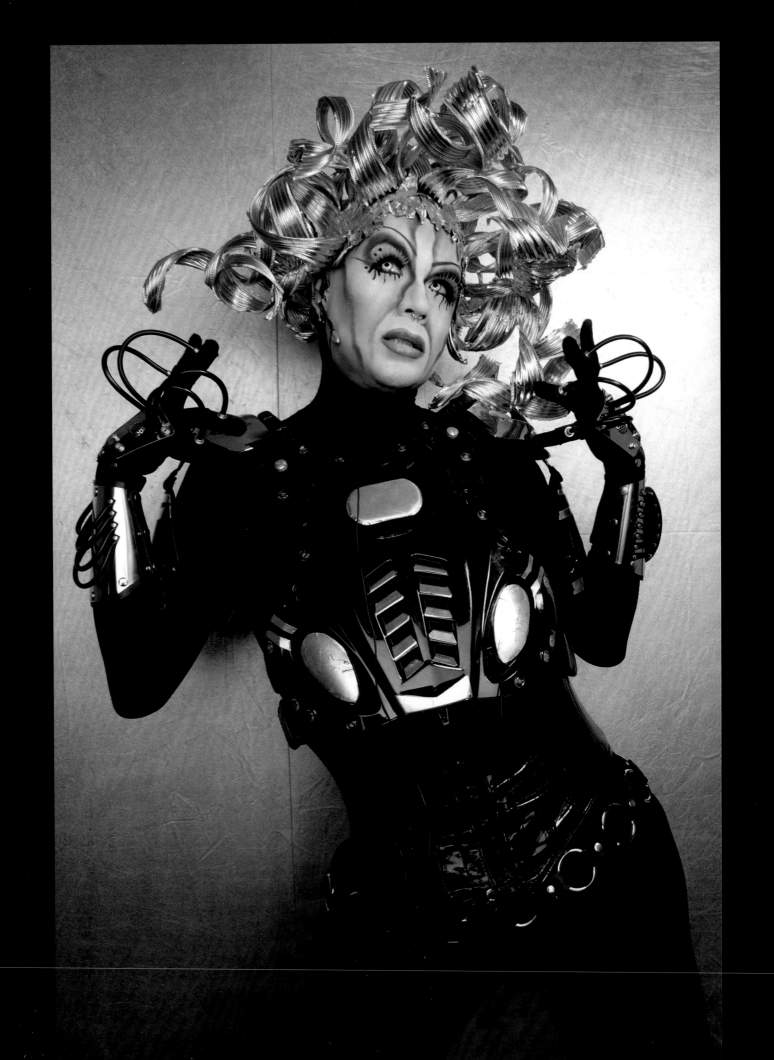

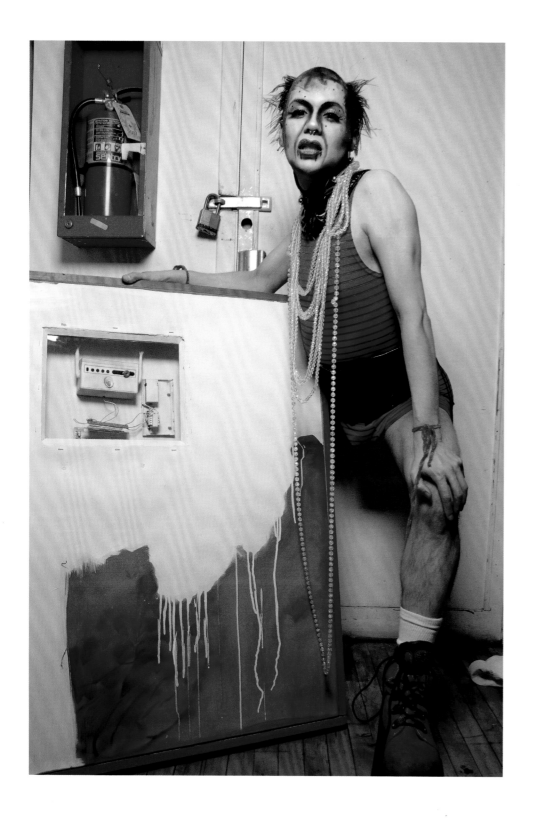
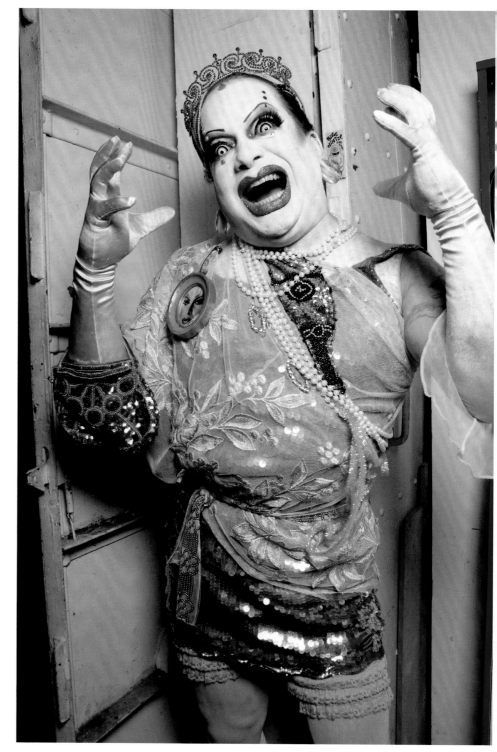

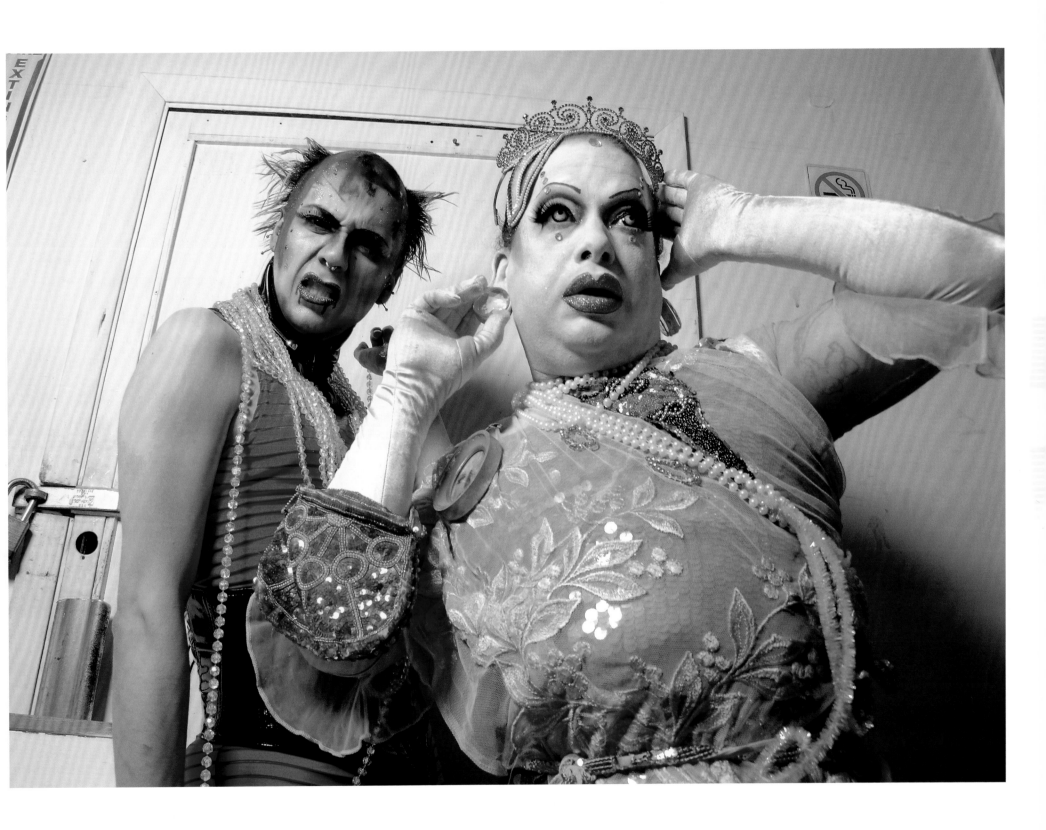

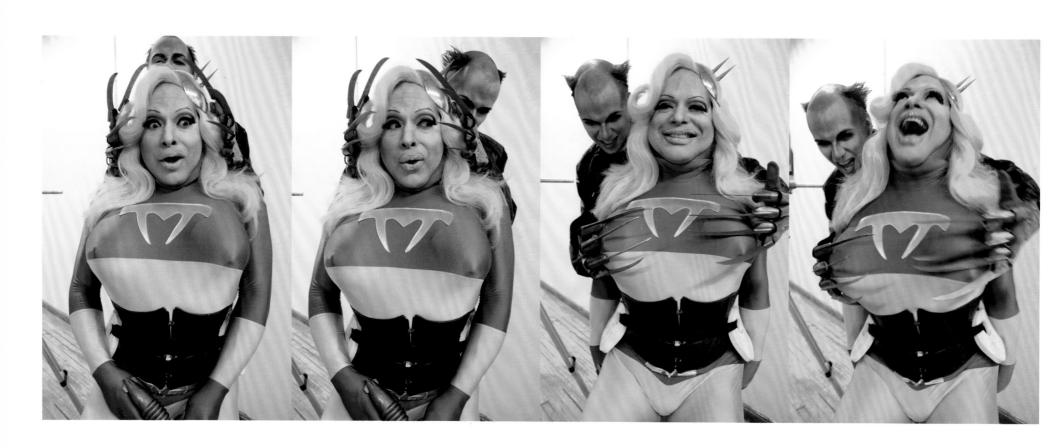

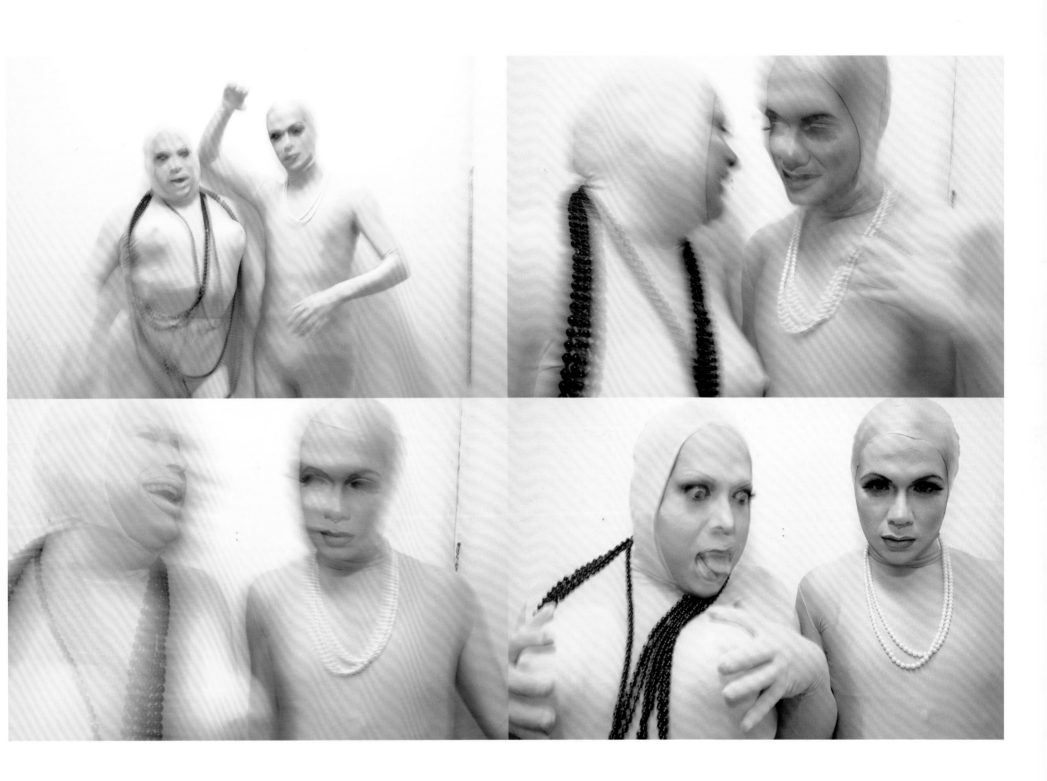

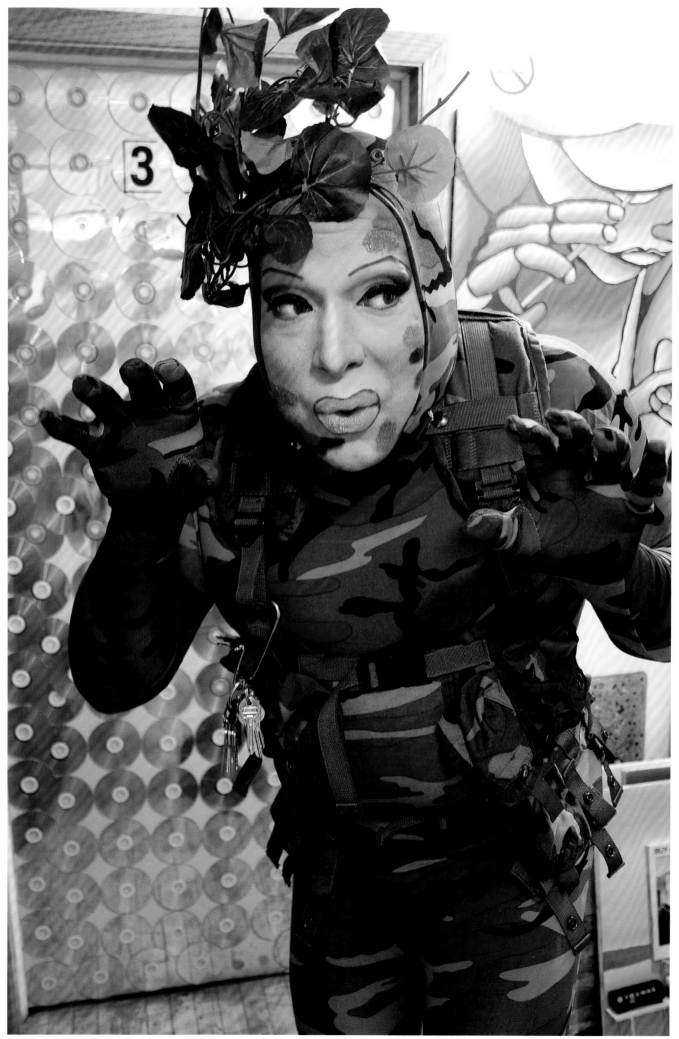

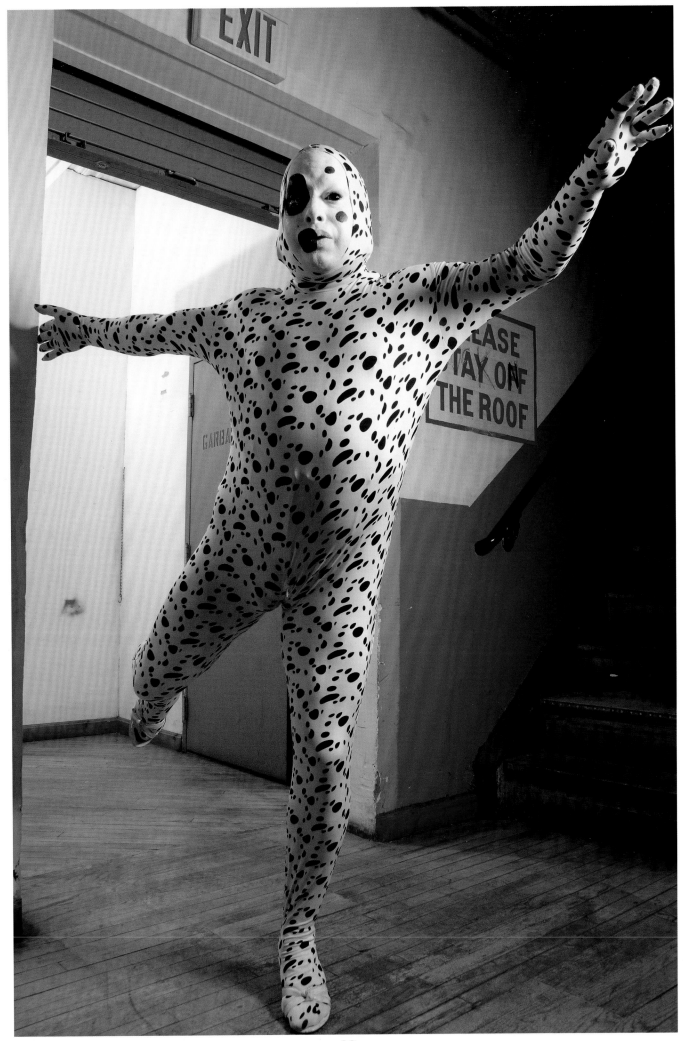

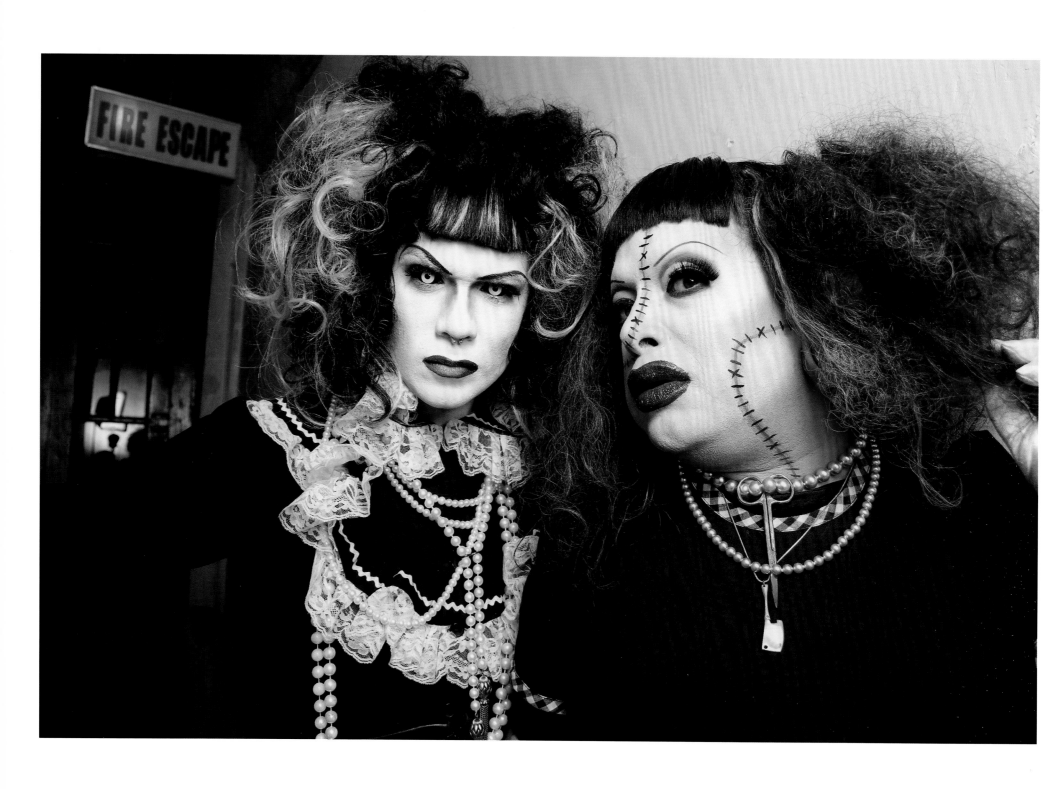

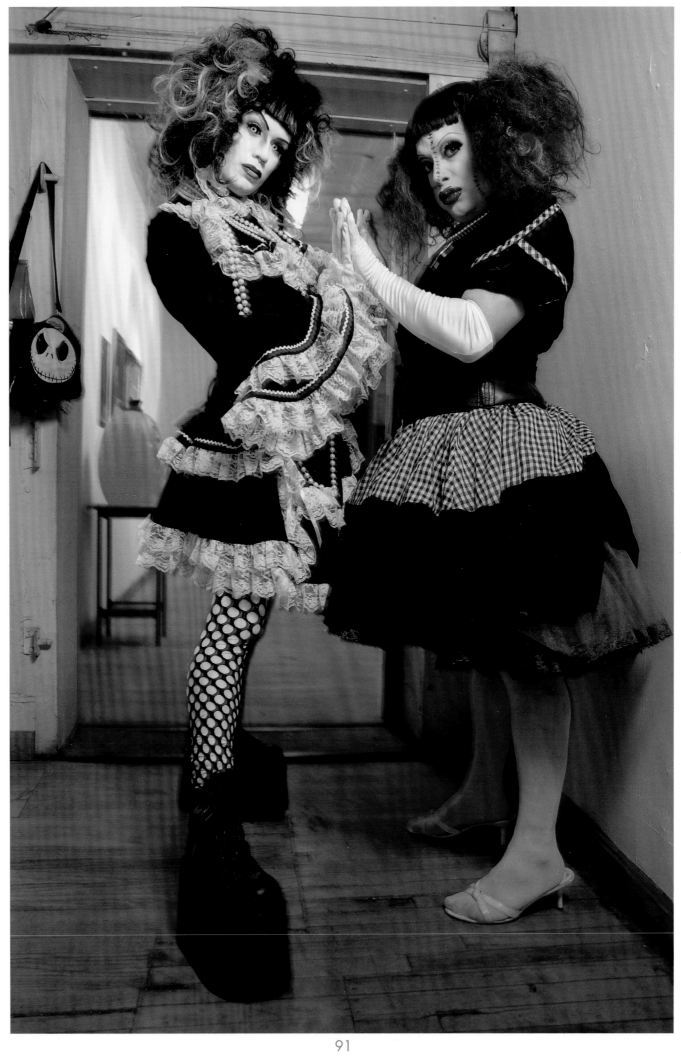

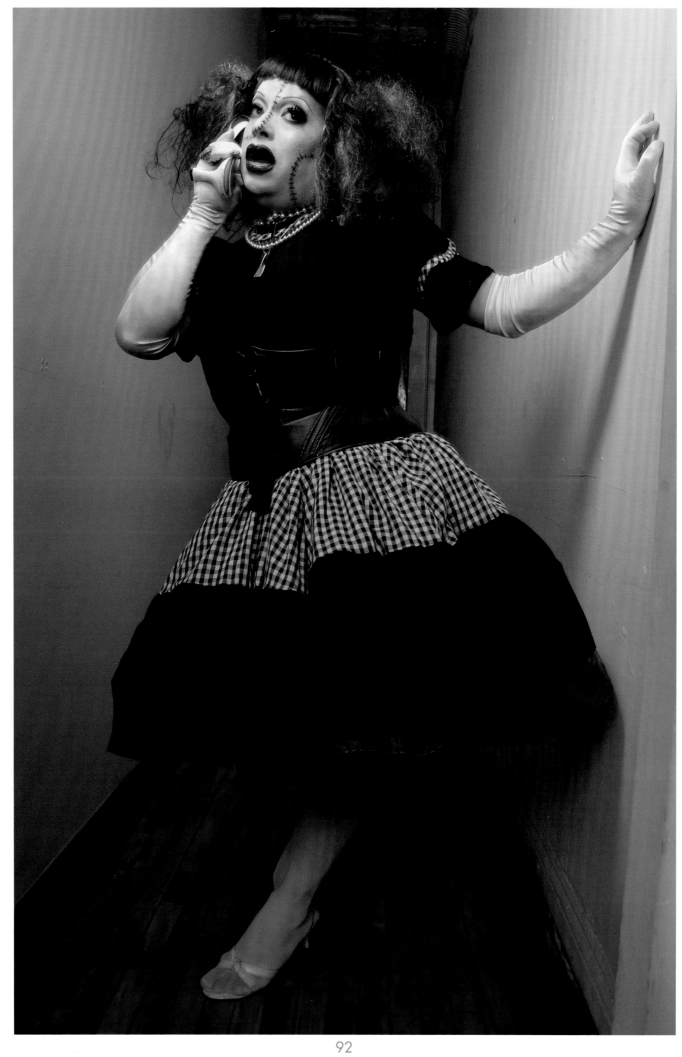

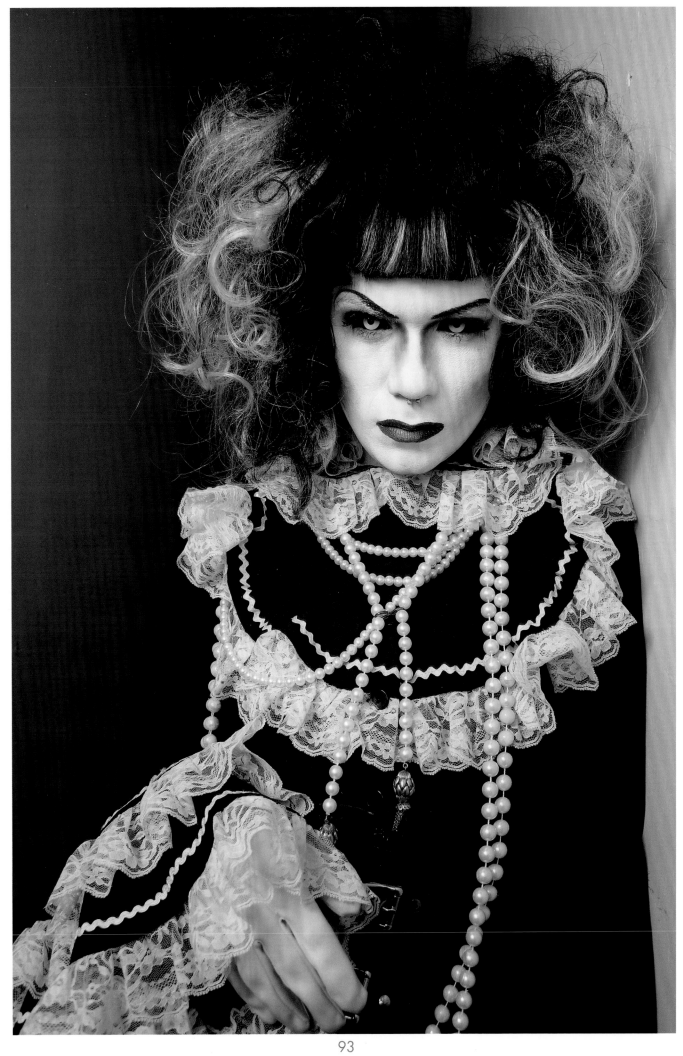

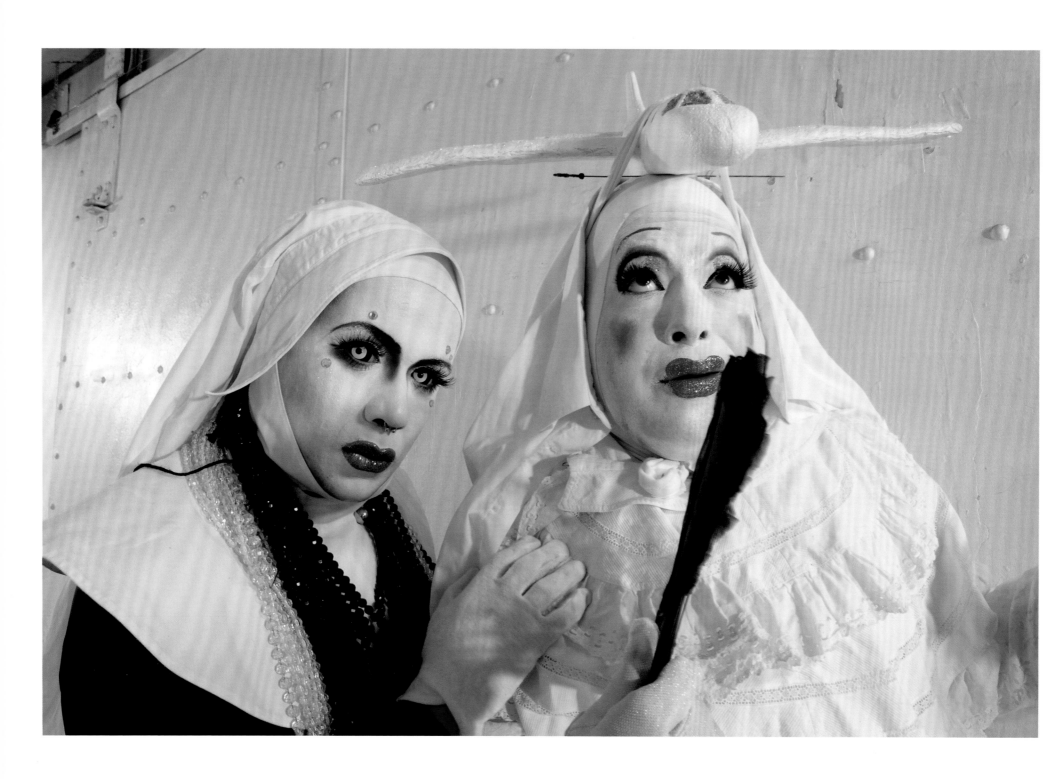

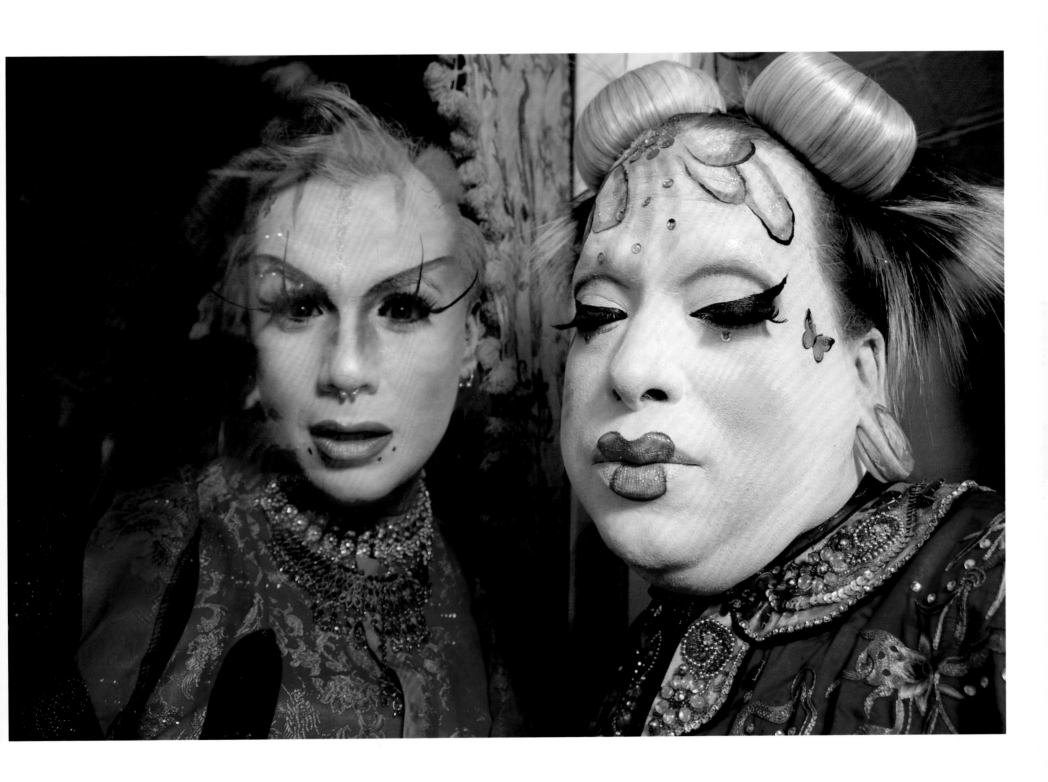

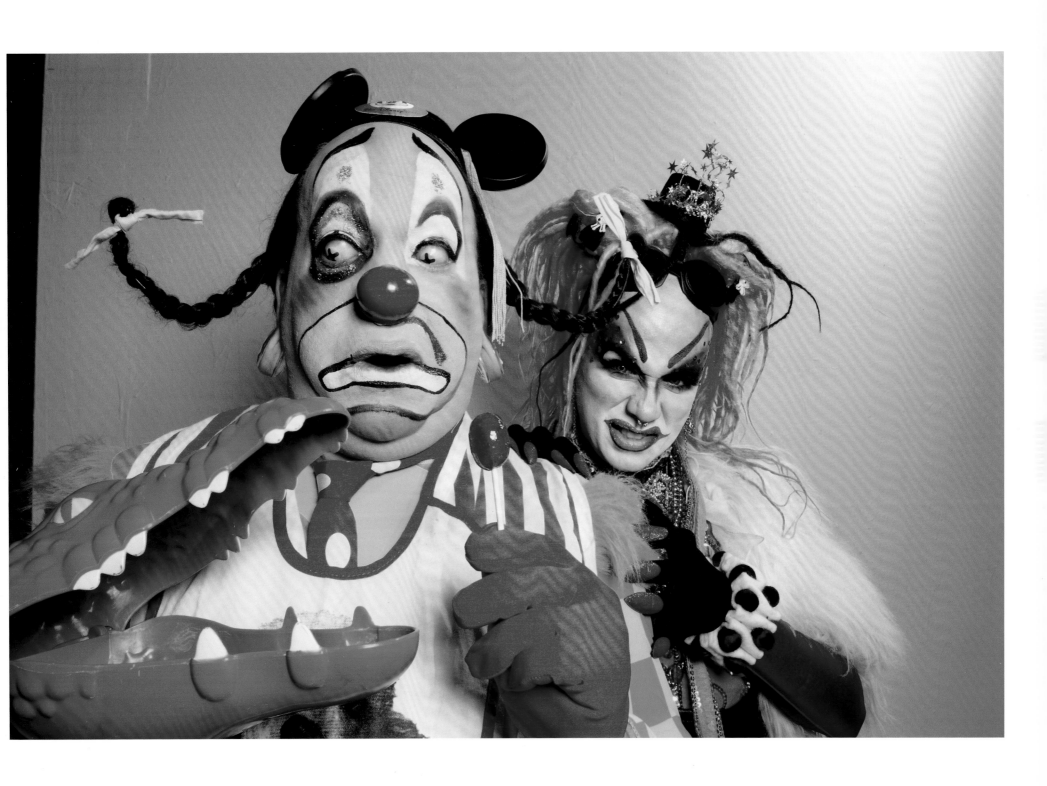

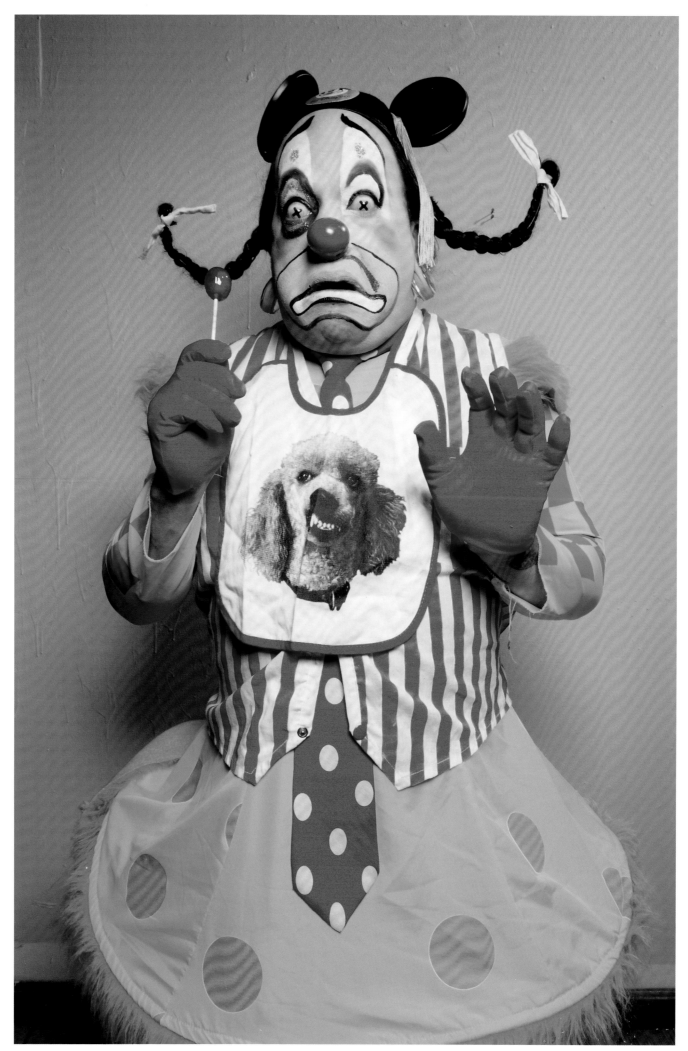

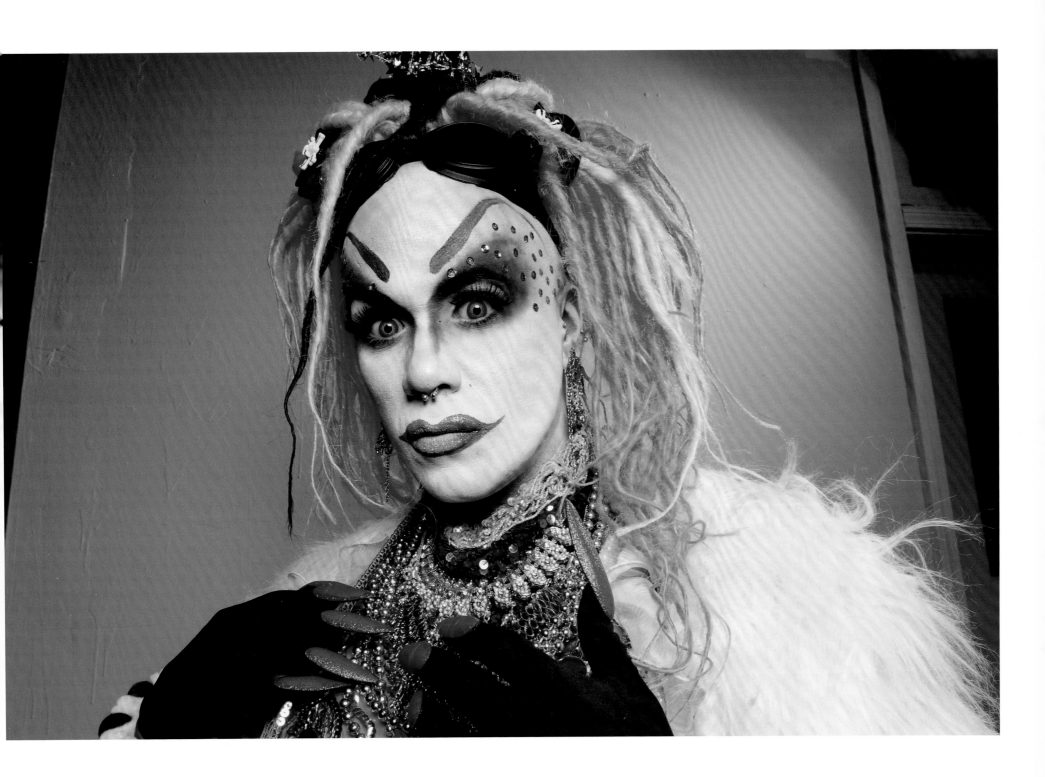

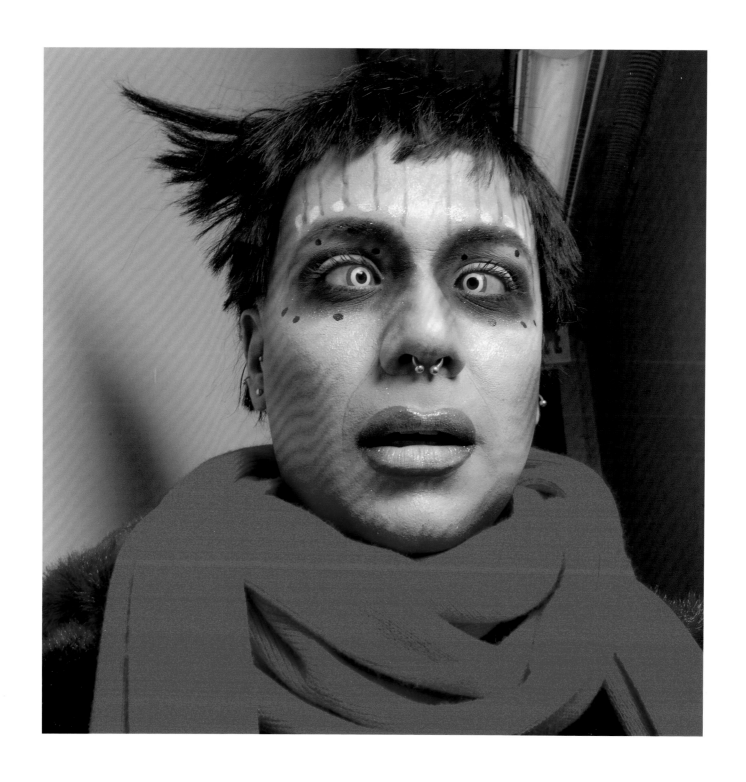

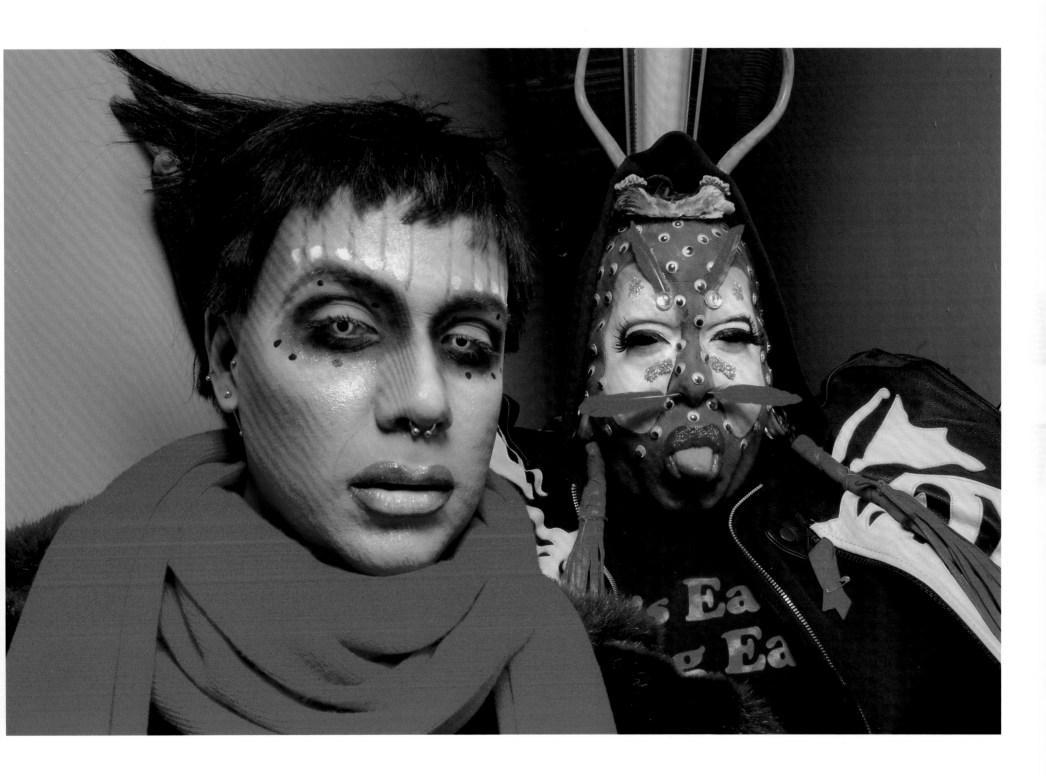

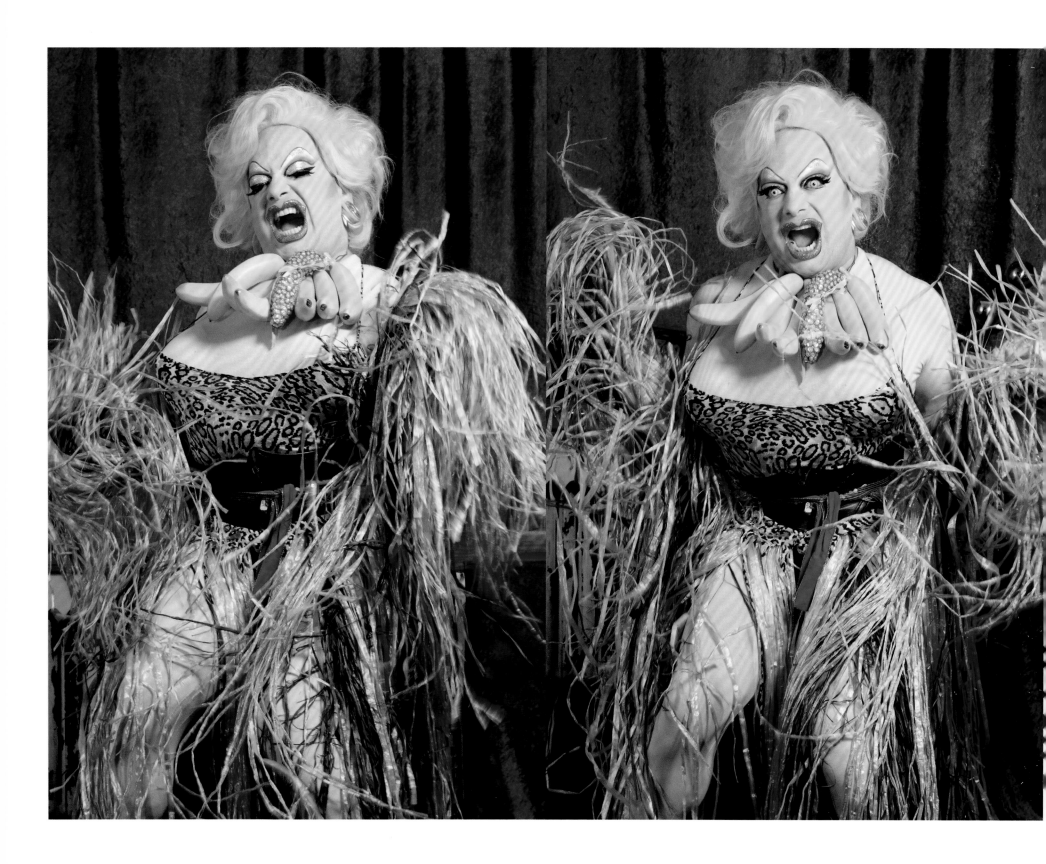

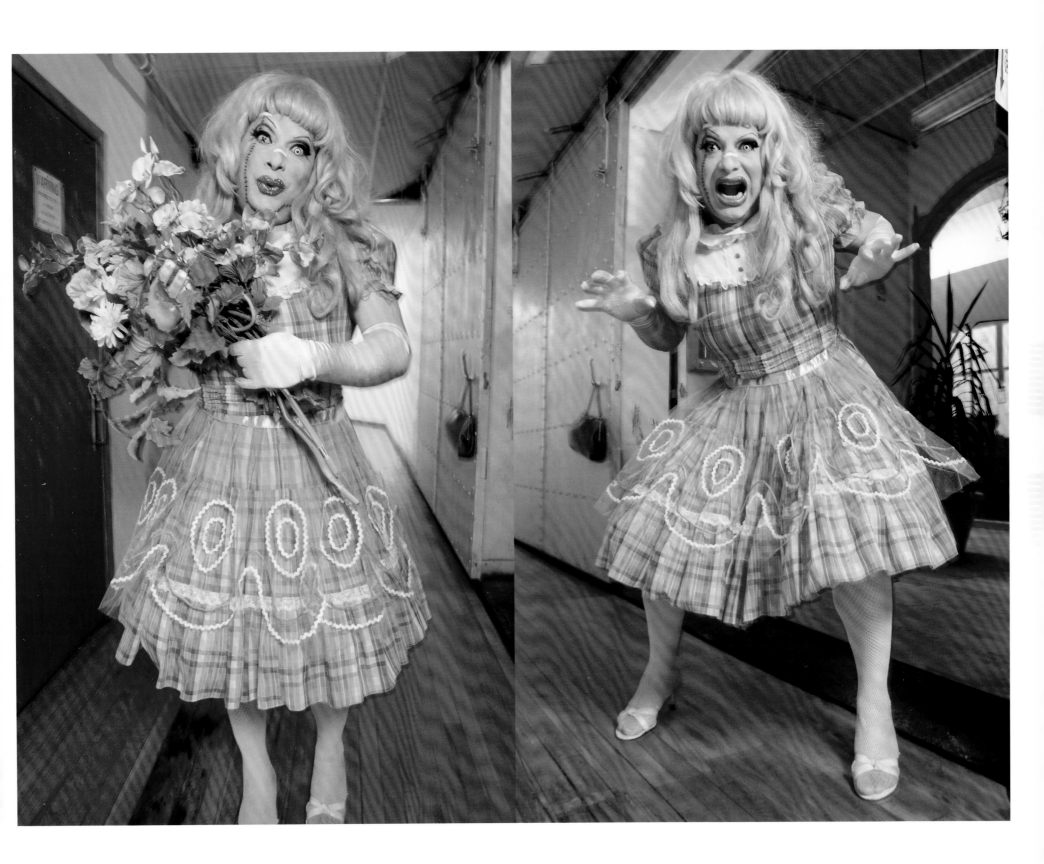

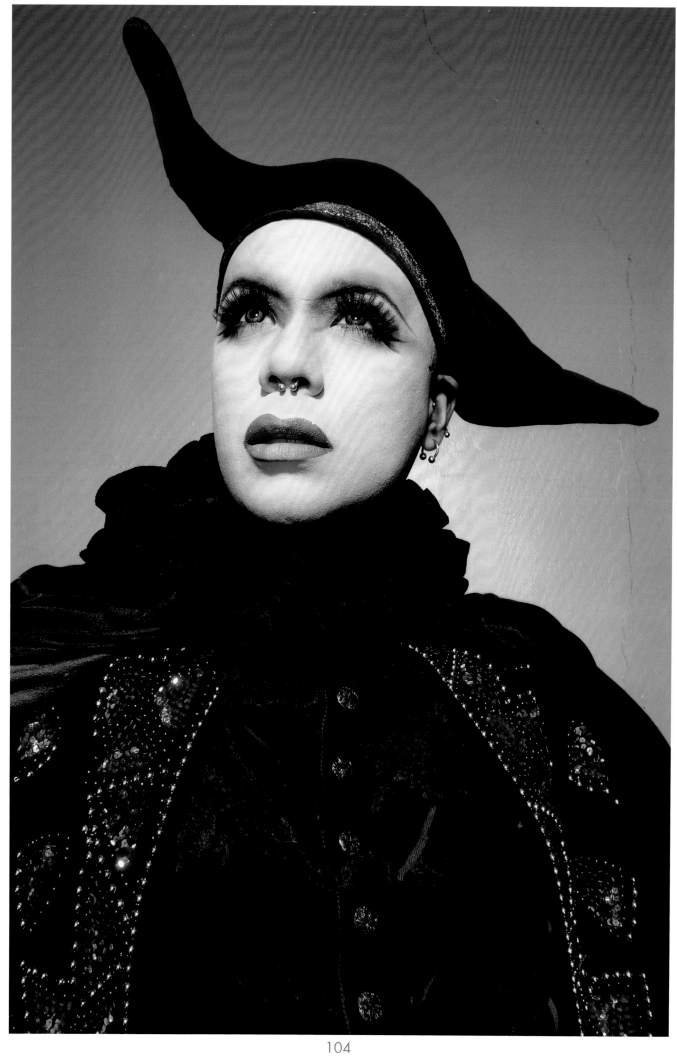

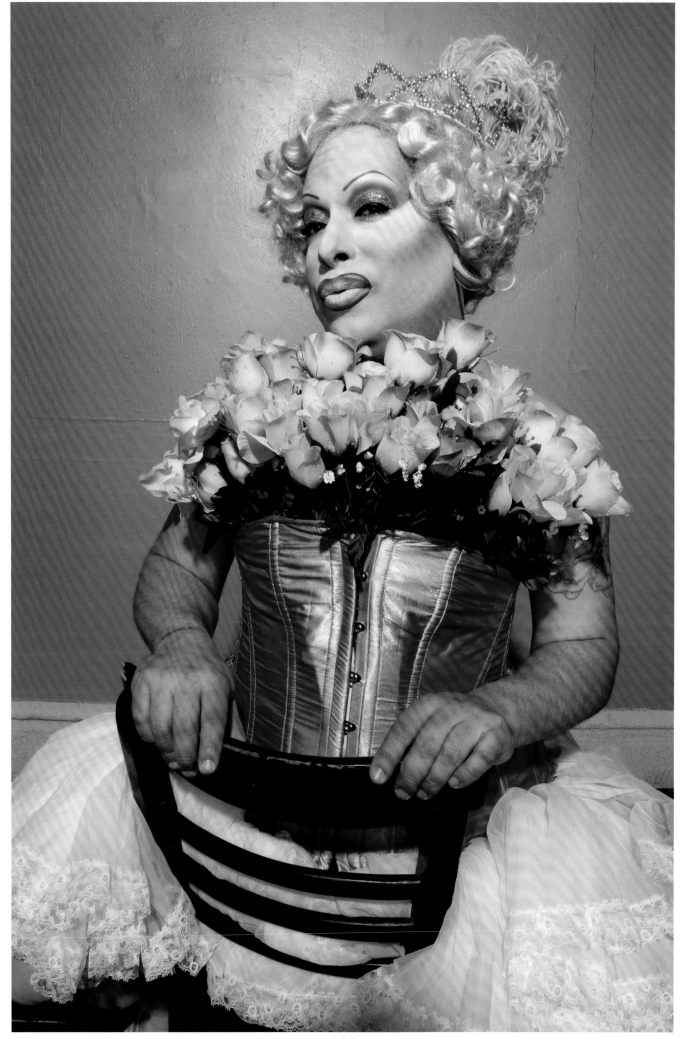

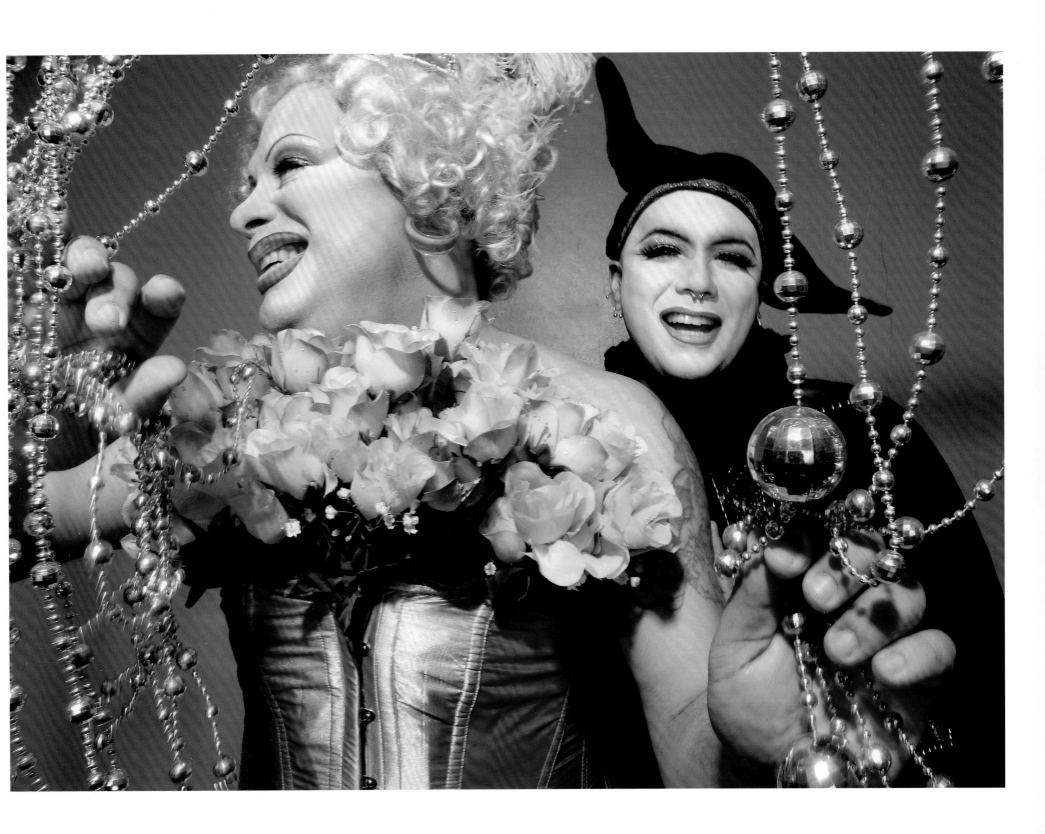

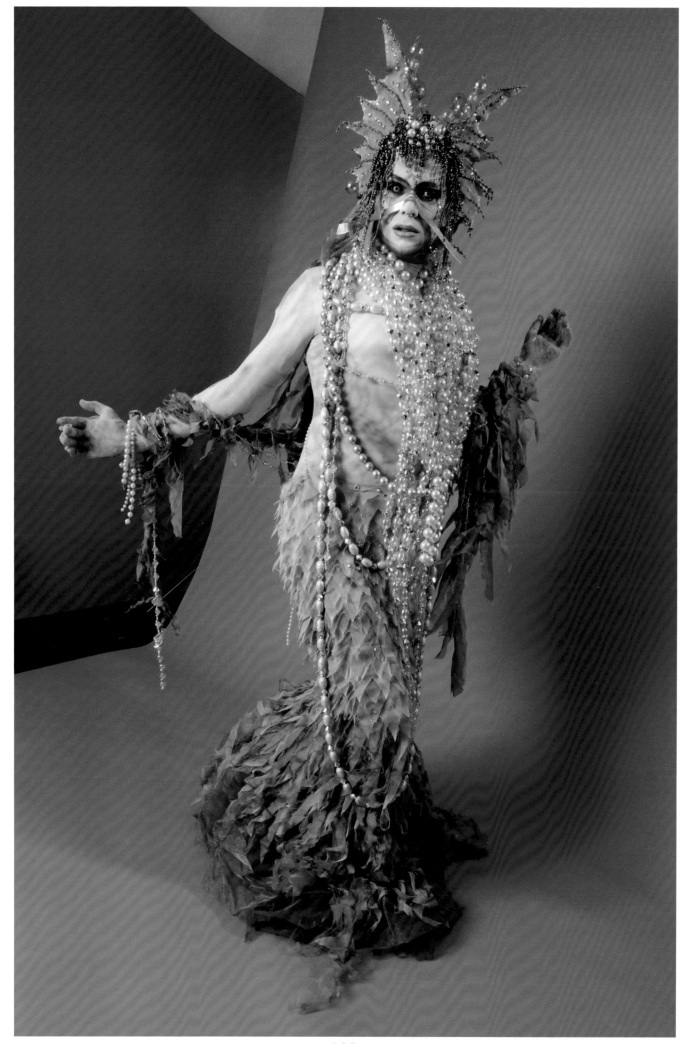

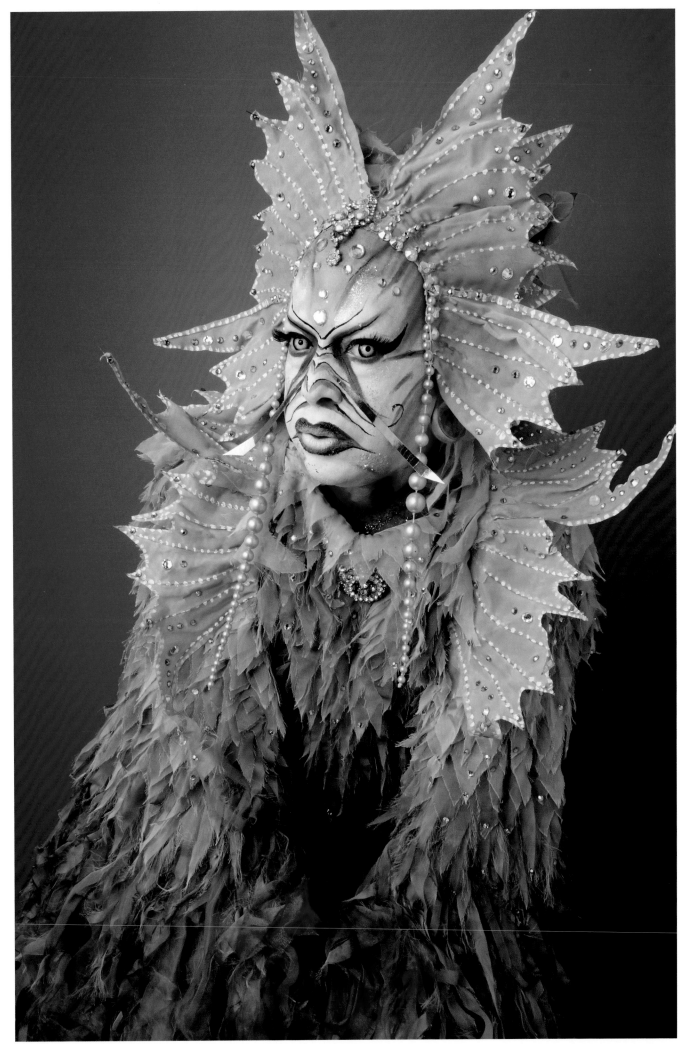

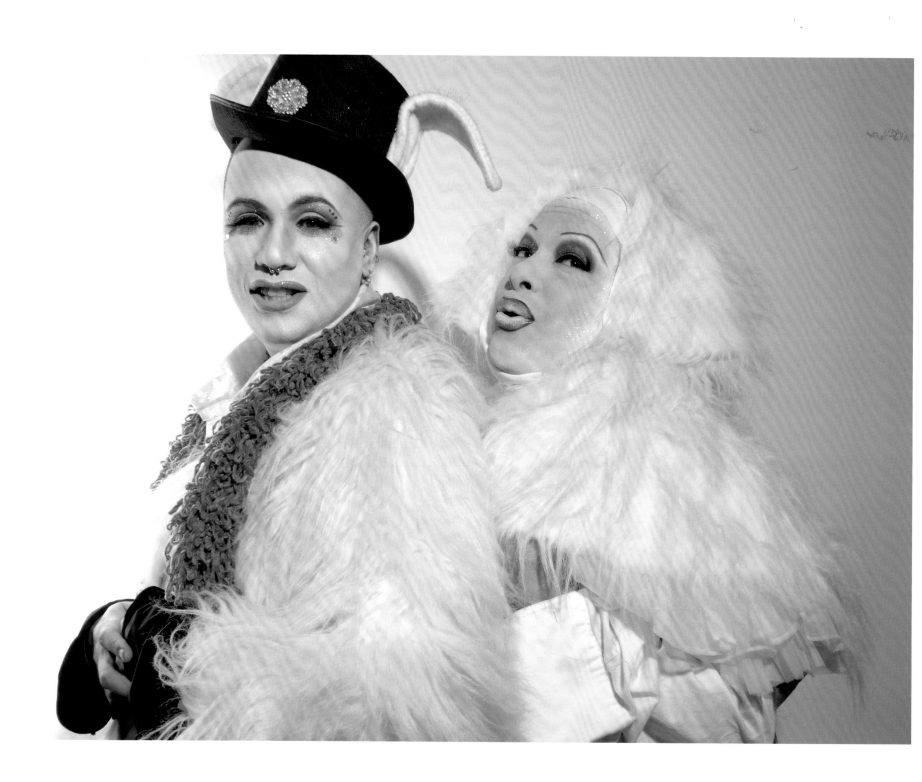

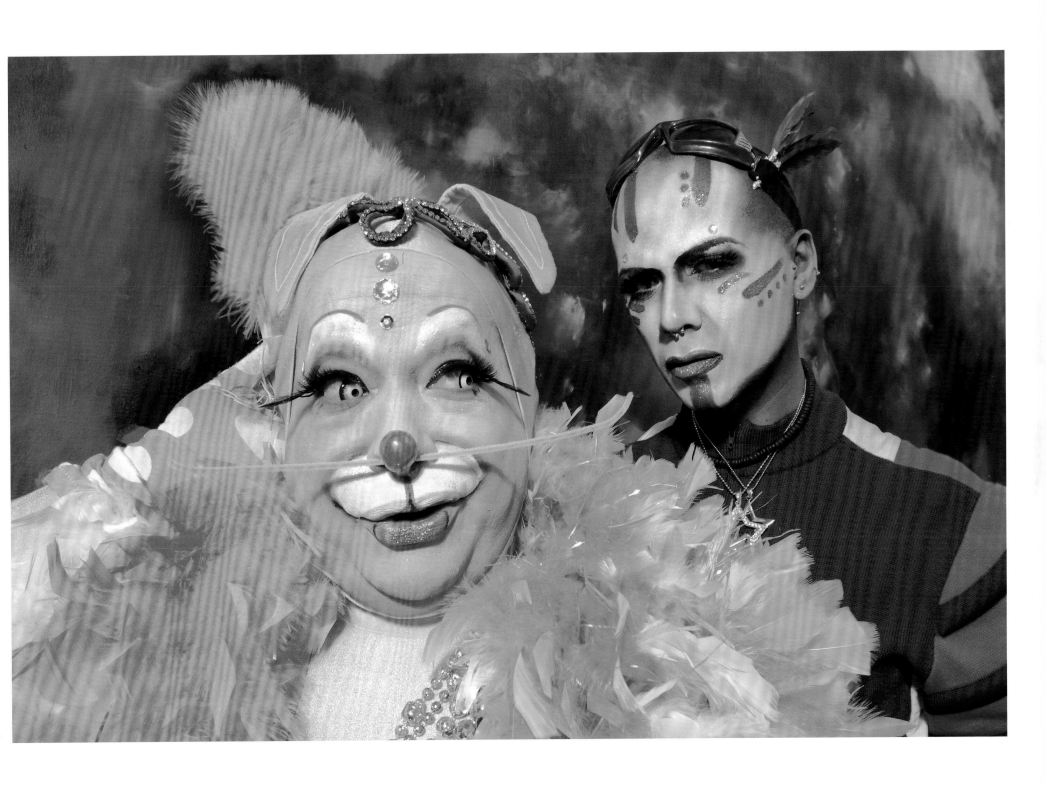

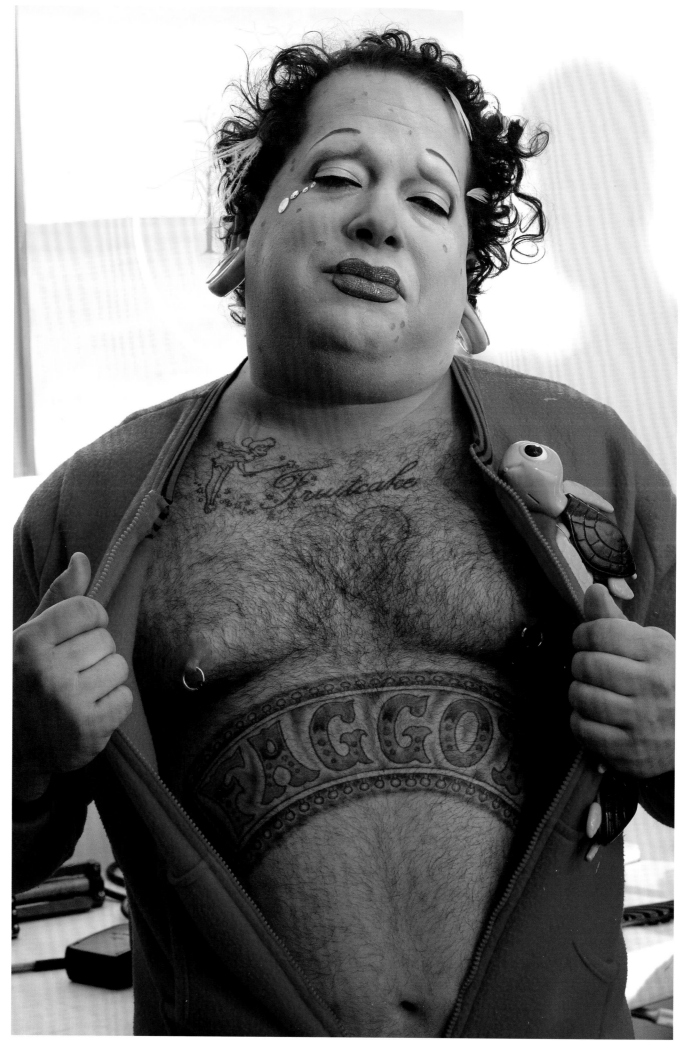

JoJo has a lot of tattoos.

He has had his body inscribed with many of the various names he's been called.

To JoJo it is a way of transmuting the pain.

He started with "Tinkerbell" and "Fruitcake." Now "Faggot" as if it is a Broadway marquee.

His favorite is "Timeless" which a friend bought him as a gift.

It is on his wrist where his watch would be, if he wore one.

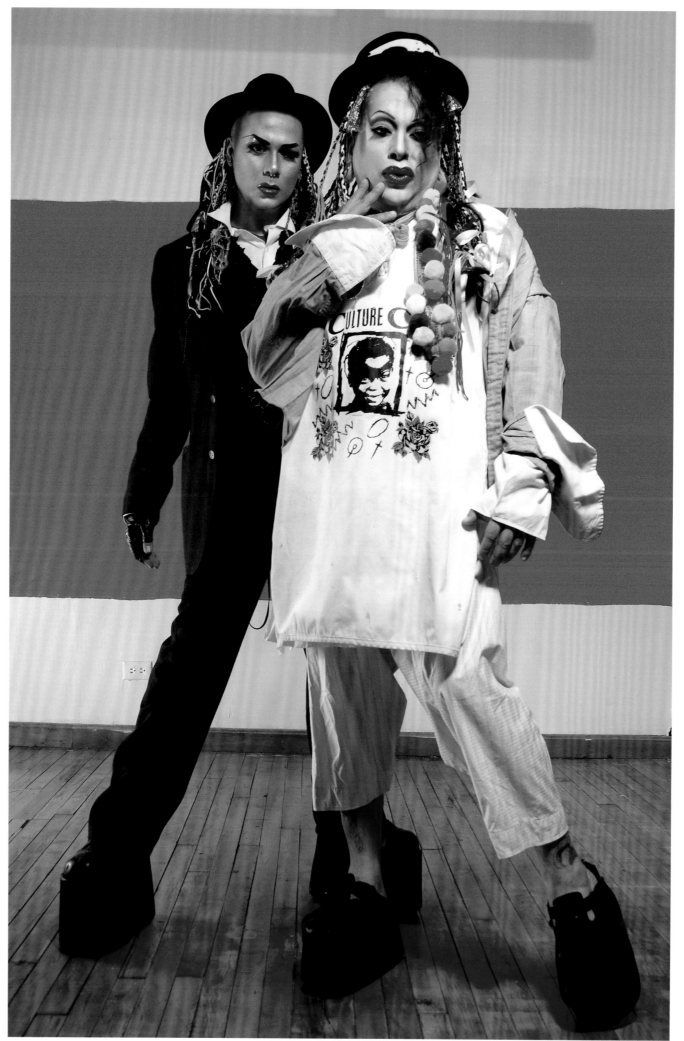

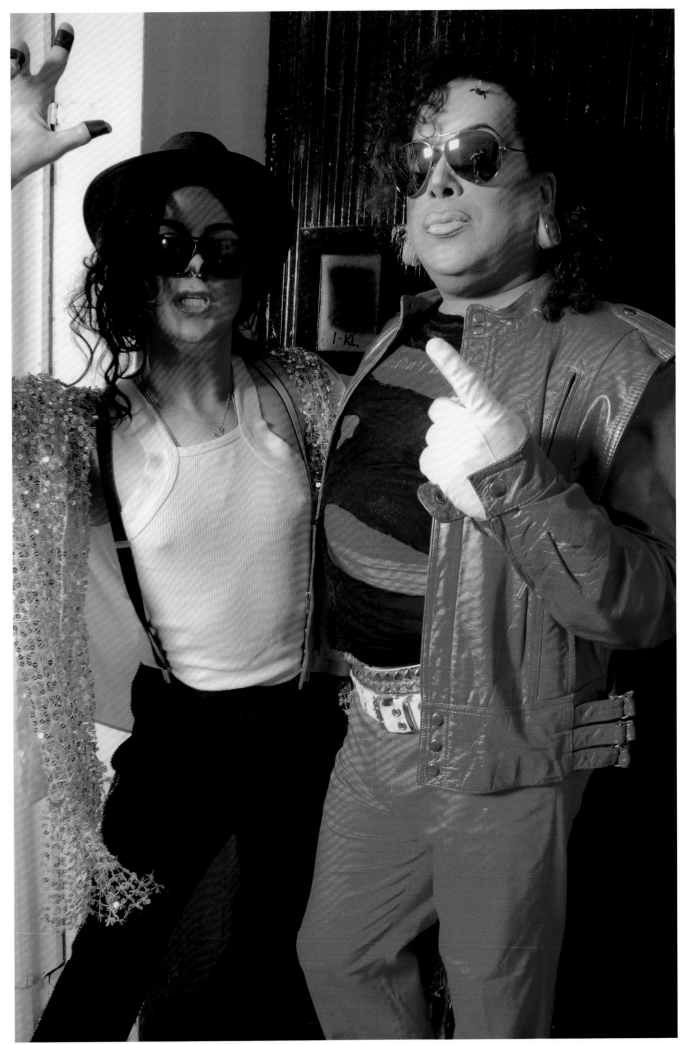

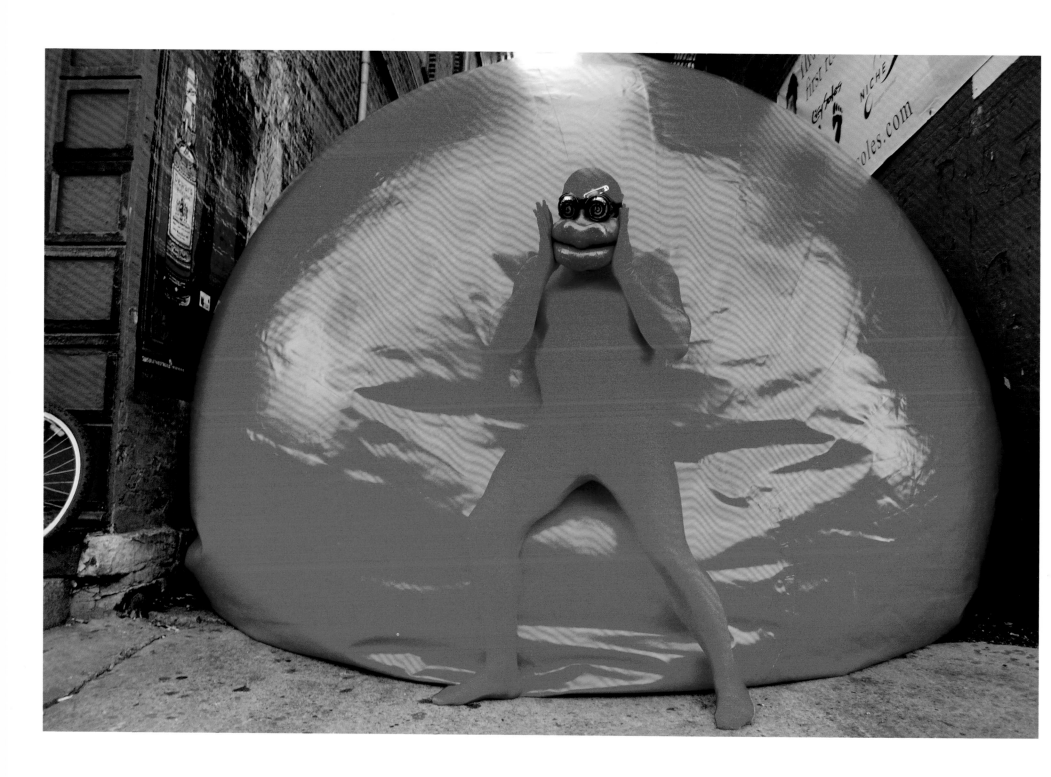

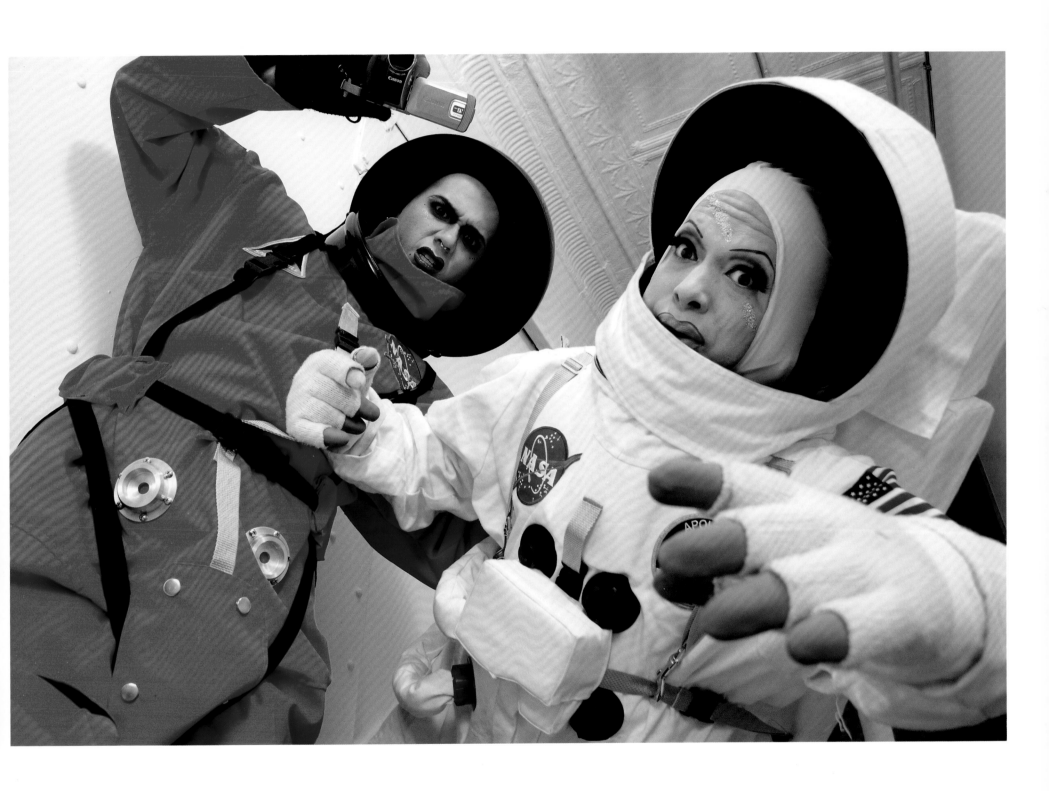

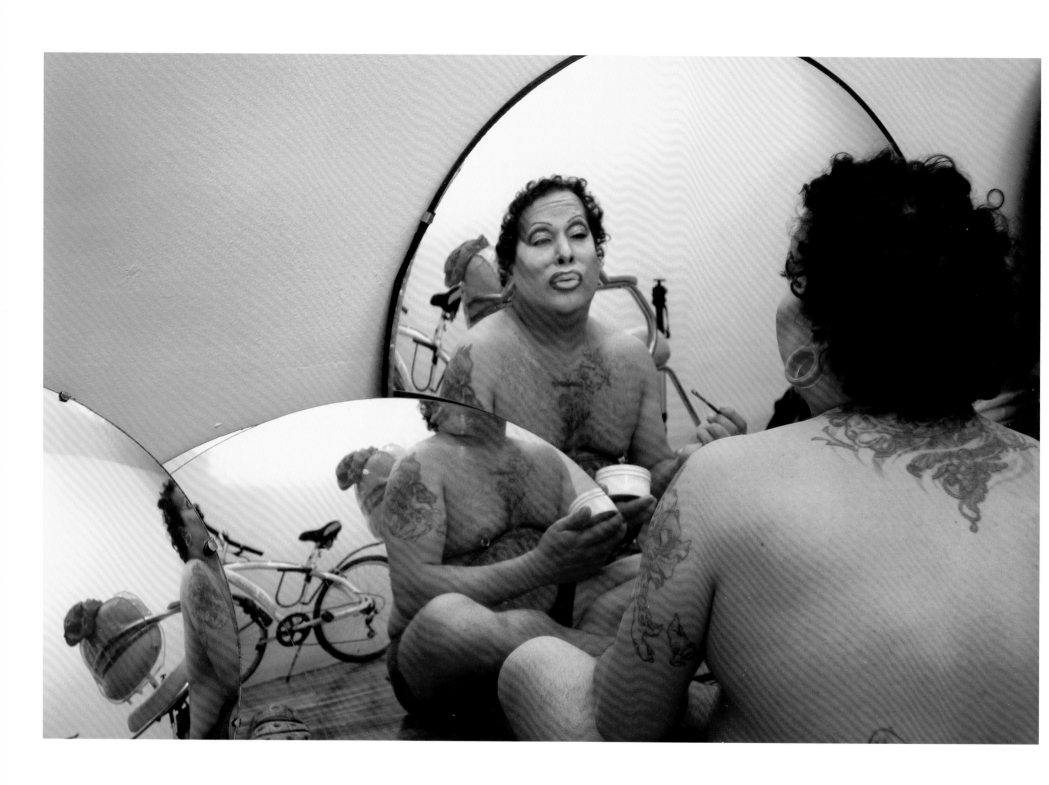

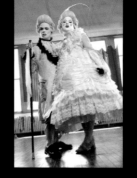

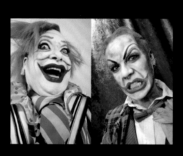

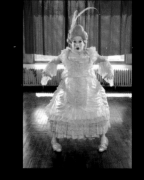

01_Soap Suds/Timeless

02_Holding Court

03_Marie Antoinette

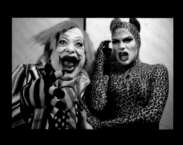

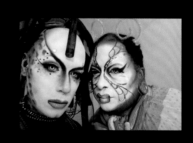

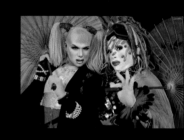

04_Super Villains

05_JoJo Joker, Sal-E Joker

06_Paper Parasols

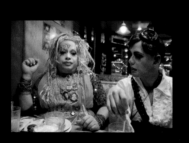

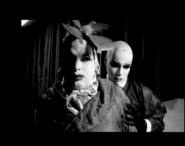

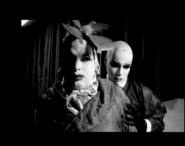

07_Breakfast at Hollywood

08_Butterflies

09_Untitled

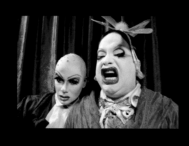

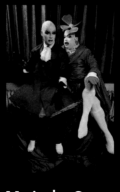

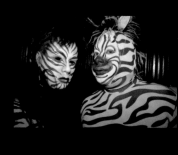

10_Strange Opera

11_At the Opera

12_Cute Zebras

INDEX

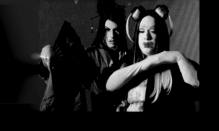

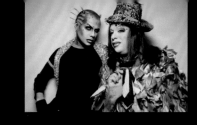

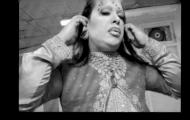

13_Geisha

14_Fashionistas

15_Untitled

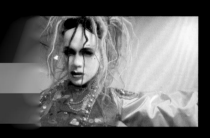

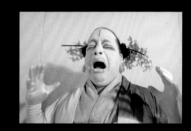

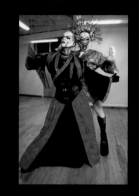

16_Untitled

17_Kabuki

18_Untitled

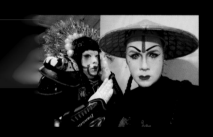

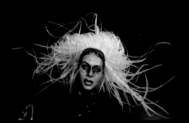

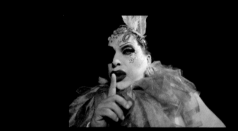

19_Untitled

20_Flying Hair

21_Shhhhhh

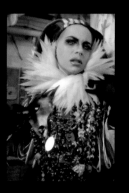

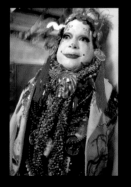

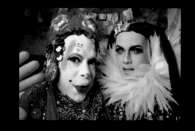

22_Sal Fat Tuesday

23_JoJo Fat Tuesday

24_Fat Tuesday

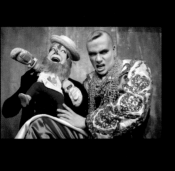

25_Leprecauns Are Real

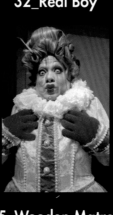

26_Snake Attack

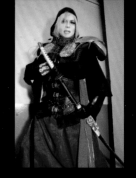

27_Untitled

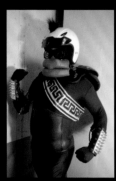

28_Untitled

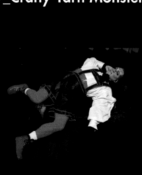

29_Crafty Yarn Monsters

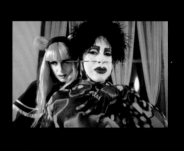

30_Ugly, at the Salon

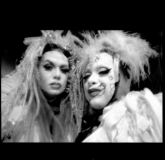

31_After Party

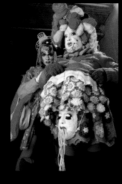

32_Real Boy

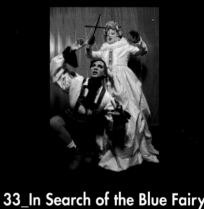

33_In Search of the Blue Fairy

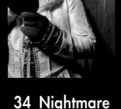

34_Nightmare

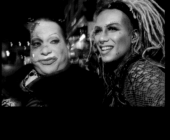

35_Wooden Matron

36_JoJo Had an Accident

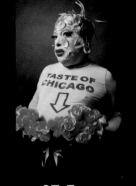

37_Taste

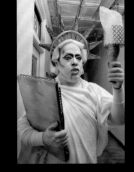

38_Shout

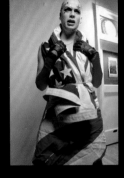

39_Lady Liberty

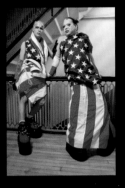

40_Election Eve, 2008

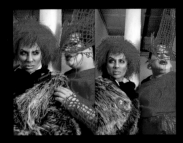

41_Red Face and String

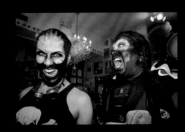

42_We Eat Babies

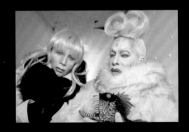

43_Atlantis

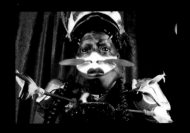

44_Scary Sal-E

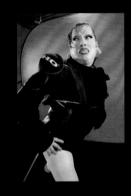

45_Wounded Warrior

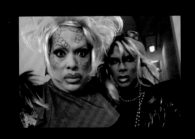

46_Mystique

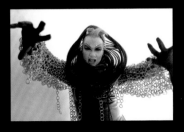

47_La Pomme Rouge

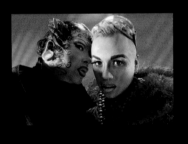

48_HO

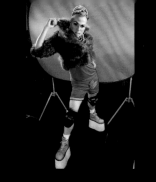

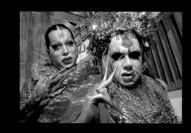

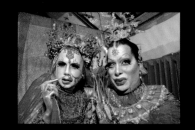

49_Heart On

50_Welcoming Fingers

51_Hindi Gods

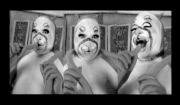

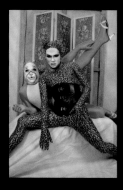

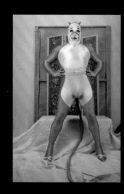

52_Cat Tails (triptych)

53_Naughty Kitties

54_Untitled

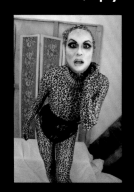

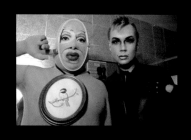

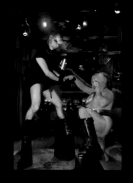

55_Untitled

56_Ladies Room

57_Dance Floor

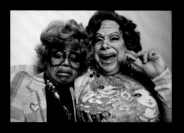

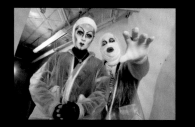

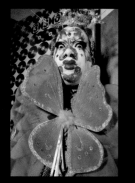

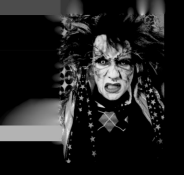

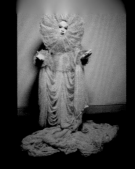

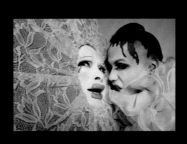

61_Untitled

62_Luna Piena

63_Night of 100 Drag Queens

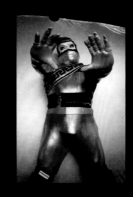

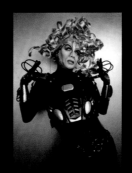

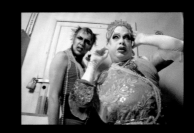

_her Nature/ Panty Party

65_Lucha Robot

66_Metallic Hair

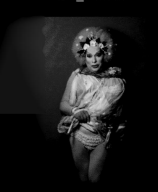

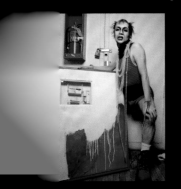

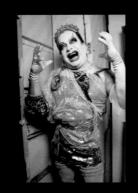

67_Untitled

68_Untitled

69_What?

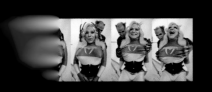

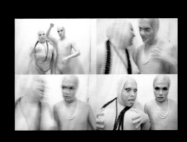

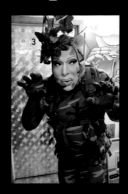

_Untitled (tetraptych)

71_Mannequins (tetraptych)

72_GI JoJo

INDEX

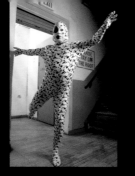
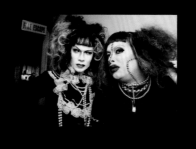
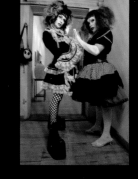
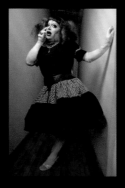
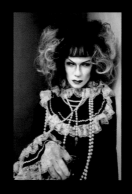
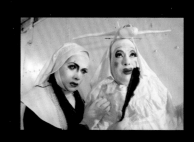
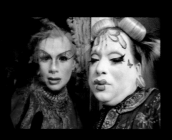
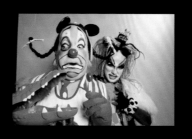
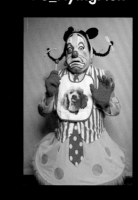
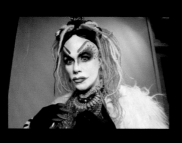
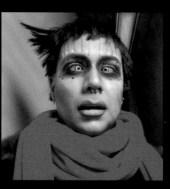
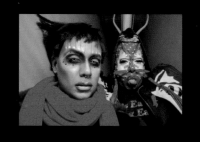
INDEX

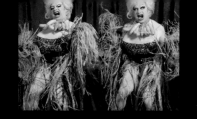
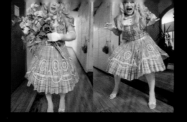
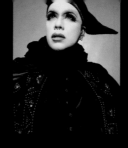

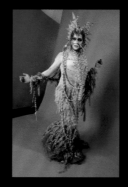

85_Divine (diptych)

86_Scary Girl (diptych)

87_Harlequin

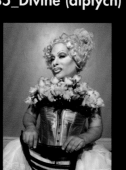
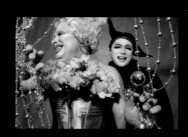
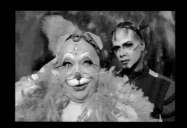

88_Blossum Bosom

89_Mardi Gras Party

90_Mermaid

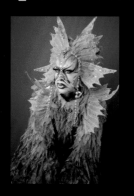
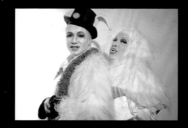
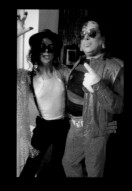

91_Merman

92_Funny Bunnies

93_Big Gay Bunny

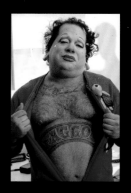
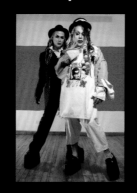
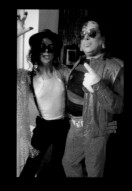

94_Sick Kid

95_Boy George Tribute

96_Peter Pan Is Dead

INDEX

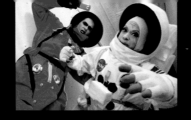

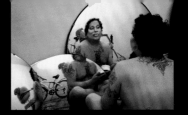

INDEX

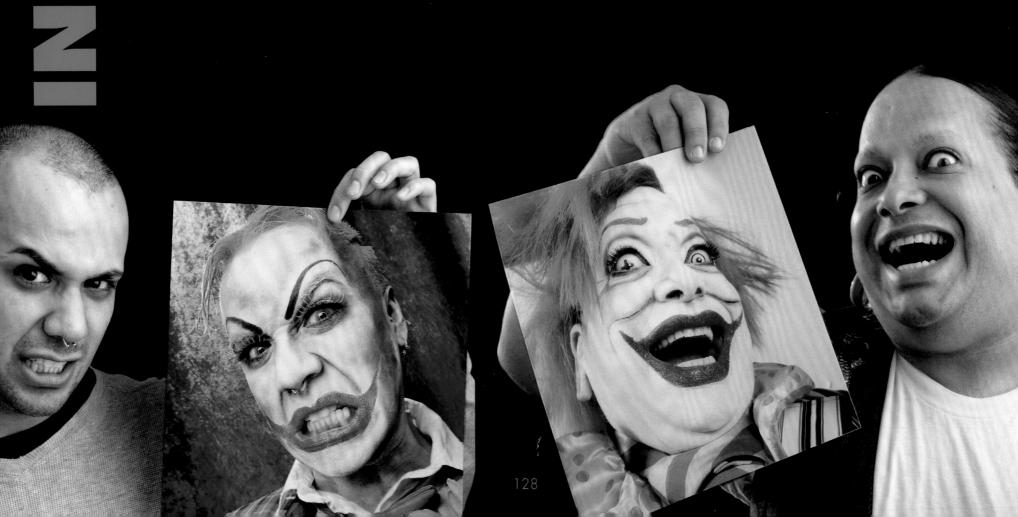

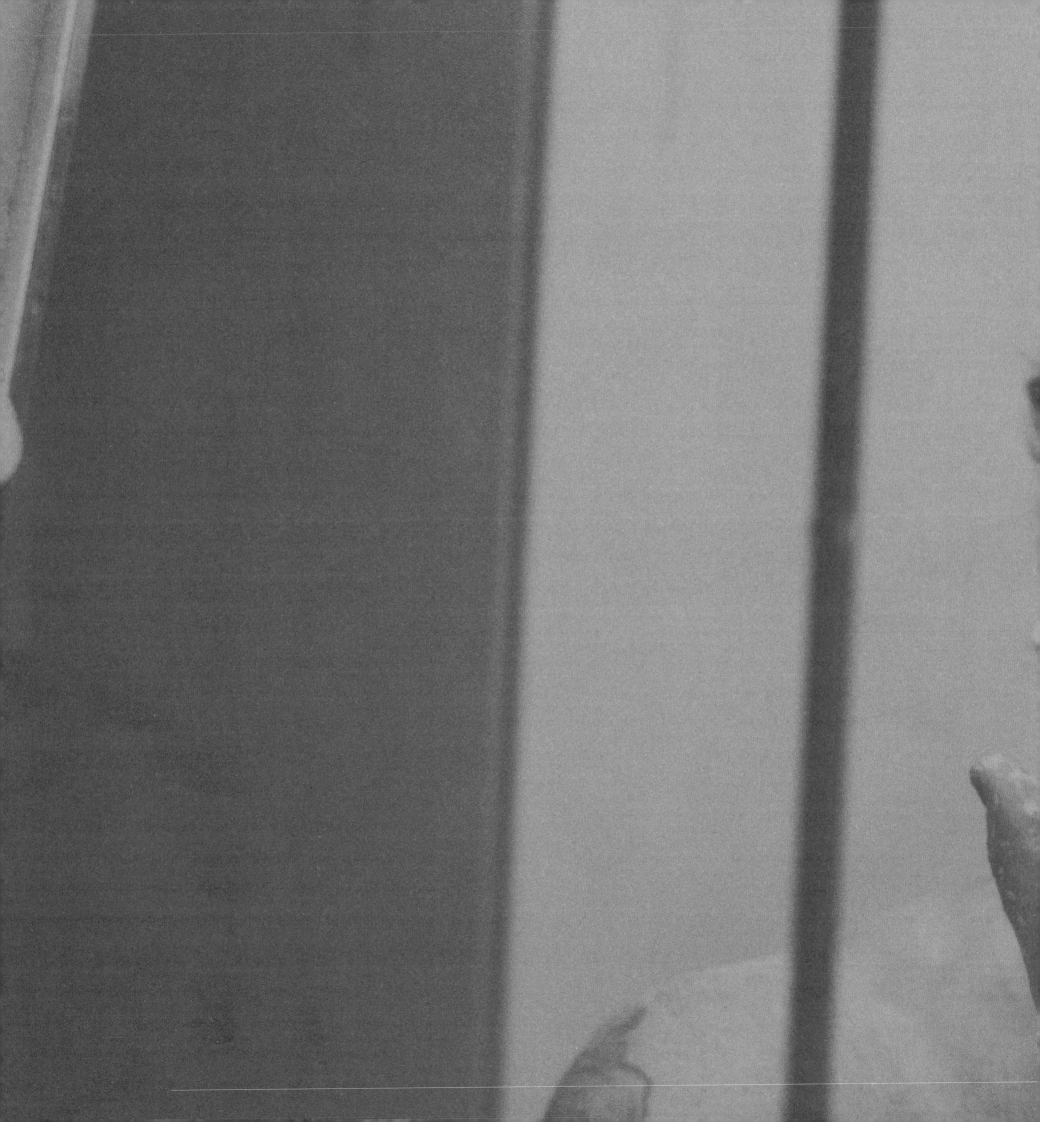